The court and country confectioner : or, the house-keeper's guide ; to a more speedy, plain, and familiar method of understanding the whole art of confectionary, pastry, distilling

Mr. Borella

The court and country confectioner : or, the house-keeper's guide ; to a more speedy, plain, and familiar method of understanding the whole art of confectionary, pastry, distilling, ... To which is added, a dissertation on the different species of fruits,
Borella, Mr.
ESTCID: T122787
Reproduction from British Library
The ingenious foreigner = Señor Borella. The final section, 'On distilling in general' has separate pagination but the register is continuous.
London : printed for G. Riley, and A. Cooke, at their Circulating Library ; J. Bell ; J. Wheble ; and C. Etherington, at York, 1770.
[2],ii,3,[1],xxiii,[1],271,[1],46p. ; 8°

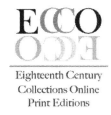

Eighteenth Century
Collections Online
Print Editions

Gale ECCO Print Editions

Relive history with *Eighteenth Century Collections Online*, now available in print for the independent historian and collector. This series includes the most significant English-language and foreign-language works printed in Great Britain during the eighteenth century, and is organized in seven different subject areas including literature and language; medicine, science, and technology; and religion and philosophy. The collection also includes thousands of important works from the Americas.

The eighteenth century has been called "The Age of Enlightenment." It was a period of rapid advance in print culture and publishing, in world exploration, and in the rapid growth of science and technology – all of which had a profound impact on the political and cultural landscape. At the end of the century the American Revolution, French Revolution and Industrial Revolution, perhaps three of the most significant events in modern history, set in motion developments that eventually dominated world political, economic, and social life.

In a groundbreaking effort, Gale initiated a revolution of its own: digitization of epic proportions to preserve these invaluable works in the largest online archive of its kind. Contributions from major world libraries constitute over 175,000 original printed works. Scanned images of the actual pages, rather than transcriptions, recreate the works *as they first appeared.*

Now for the first time, these high-quality digital scans of original works are available via print-on-demand, making them readily accessible to libraries, students, independent scholars, and readers of all ages.

For our initial release we have created seven robust collections to form one the world's most comprehensive catalogs of 18th century works.

Initial Gale ECCO Print Editions collections include:

History and Geography
Rich in titles on English life and social history, this collection spans the world as it was known to eighteenth-century historians and explorers. Titles include a wealth of travel accounts and diaries, histories of nations from throughout the world, and maps and charts of a world that was still being discovered. Students of the War of American Independence will find fascinating accounts from the British side of conflict.

Social Science
Delve into what it was like to live during the eighteenth century by reading the first-hand accounts of everyday people, including city dwellers and farmers, businessmen and bankers, artisans and merchants, artists and their patrons, politicians and their constituents. Original texts make the American, French, and Industrial revolutions vividly contemporary.

Medicine, Science and Technology
Medical theory and practice of the 1700s developed rapidly, as is evidenced by the extensive collection, which includes descriptions of diseases, their conditions, and treatments. Books on science and technology, agriculture, military technology, natural philosophy, even cookbooks, are all contained here.

Literature and Language
Western literary study flows out of eighteenth-century works by Alexander Pope, Daniel Defoe, Henry Fielding, Frances Burney, Denis Diderot, Johann Gottfried Herder, Johann Wolfgang von Goethe, and others. Experience the birth of the modern novel, or compare the development of language using dictionaries and grammar discourses.

Religion and Philosophy
The Age of Enlightenment profoundly enriched religious and philosophical understanding and continues to influence present-day thinking. Works collected here include masterpieces by David Hume, Immanuel Kant, and Jean-Jacques Rousseau, as well as religious sermons and moral debates on the issues of the day, such as the slave trade. The Age of Reason saw conflict between Protestantism and Catholicism transformed into one between faith and logic -- a debate that continues in the twenty-first century.

Law and Reference
This collection reveals the history of English common law and Empire law in a vastly changing world of British expansion. Dominating the legal field is the *Commentaries of the Law of England* by Sir William Blackstone, which first appeared in 1765. Reference works such as almanacs and catalogues continue to educate us by revealing the day-to-day workings of society.

Fine Arts
The eighteenth-century fascination with Greek and Roman antiquity followed the systematic excavation of the ruins at Pompeii and Herculaneum in southern Italy; and after 1750 a neoclassical style dominated all artistic fields. The titles here trace developments in mostly English-language works on painting, sculpture, architecture, music, theater, and other disciplines. Instructional works on musical instruments, catalogs of art objects, comic operas, and more are also included.

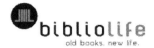

The BiblioLife Network

This project was made possible in part by the BiblioLife Network (BLN), a project aimed at addressing some of the huge challenges facing book preservationists around the world. The BLN includes libraries, library networks, archives, subject matter experts, online communities and library service providers. We believe every book ever published should be available as a high-quality print reproduction; printed on-demand anywhere in the world. This insures the ongoing accessibility of the content and helps generate sustainable revenue for the libraries and organizations that work to preserve these important materials.

The following book is in the "public domain" and represents an authentic reproduction of the text as printed by the original publisher. While we have attempted to accurately maintain the integrity of the original work, there are sometimes problems with the original work or the micro-film from which the books were digitized. This can result in minor errors in reproduction. Possible imperfections include missing and blurred pages, poor pictures, markings and other reproduction issues beyond our control. Because this work is culturally important, we have made it available as part of our commitment to protecting, preserving, and promoting the world's literature.

GUIDE TO FOLD-OUTS MAPS and OVERSIZED IMAGES

The book you are reading was digitized from microfilm captured over the past thirty to forty years. Years after the creation of the original microfilm, the book was converted to digital files and made available in an online database.

In an online database, page images do not need to conform to the size restrictions found in a printed book. When converting these images back into a printed bound book, the page sizes are standardized in ways that maintain the detail of the original. For large images, such as fold-out maps, the original page image is split into two or more pages

Guidelines used to determine how to split the page image follows:

- Some images are split vertically; large images require vertical and horizontal splits.
- For horizontal splits, the content is split left to right.
- For vertical splits, the content is split from top to bottom.
- For both vertical and horizontal splits, the image is processed from top left to bottom right.

THE COURT AND COUNTRY CONFECTIONER:

OR, THE HOUSE-KEEPER'S GUIDE;

To a more speedy, plain, and familiar method of understanding the whole art of confectionary, pastry, distilling, and the making of fine flavoured English wines from all kinds of fruits, herbs, and flowers; comprehending near four hundred and fifty easy and practical receipts, never before made known.

PARTICULARLY,

PRESERVING.
CANDYING
ICING
TRANSPARENT MARMALADE,
ORANGE,
PINE APPLE,
PISTACHIO, and other Rich Creams
CARAMEL.
PASTILS
BOMBOONS.

PUFF, SPUN, and FRUIT-PASTES
LIGHT BISCUITS.
PUFFS.
RICH SEED-CAKES.
CUSTARDS.
SYLLABUBS.
FLUMMERIES.
TRIFLES. WHIPS. FRUITS, and other JELLIES.
PICKLES, &c. &c.

ALSO

New and easy directions for clarifying the different degrees of sugar, together with several bills of fare of deserts for private gentlemen's families.

To which is added,

A dissertation on the different species of fruits, and the art of distilling simple waters, cordials, perfumed oils, and essences.

By an INGENIOUS FOREIGNER, now Head confectioner to the Spanish Ambassador in England.

LONDON.

Printed for G. RILEY, and A. COOKE, at their Circulating Library, *Queen Street, Berkley Square*; J BELL, near *Exeter-Exchange*, in the *Strand*; J. WHEBLE, at No. 20. *Pater-noster-row*; and C. ETHERINGTON, at *York*.

M.DCC.LXX.

DEDICATION

TO THE

LADIES

OF

GREAT BRITAIN.

IT may be said, dedications are appendages that ought only to accompany works of a more important nature; yet as there are many, very many ladies in this kingdom, whose shining example, both in public and private life, render them

the

the most amiable patterns of household œconomy, and who think it no speck on their characters, in descending to recommend to their domestics, whatsoever may be either useful or ornamental at their table; the following easy and practical receipts will, it is hoped, obtain their approbation and patronage.

THE AUTHOR's ADDRESS TO THE HOUSE-KEEPERS OF GREAT-BRITAIN.

AS a writer, I have little or no pretention, nor were I at all inclinable, to let any apology accompany the following sheets; well knowing, that the most elaborate illustration that could be thrown upon such a subject, would not

add

add one tittle to the value of such a work. Nay, on the other hand, it might be a means to draw upon me the resentment of many master confectioners whom I have reason to believe, will be a good deal irritated; for like the dyers and distillers, their whole art may be said to consist in being known to none but its professors; and while it must be owned, that, in noblemen's families the assistance of a confectioner on many occasions, cannot be avoided; yet, after many years experience in that capacity abroad, together with having lived several years in England, in some of the most distinguished families as confectioner. I say, after so many years experience, it

it

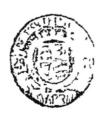

is not without some hopes of success, when I shew that there are few or no receipts in confectionary and distilling but what may be easily and successfully practised by the English house-keeper.

CONTENTS.

BOMBOONS. Page.

——— ALMONDS Bitter　36
——— Coffee cream　37
——— Nut　34
——— Orange flower　38

Baking of Biscuits, observations on　259

Biscuits Blowed　234
——— Chocolate　235
——— Diet　233
——— Fruit　236

Another of Preserved or Dried.　238

——— French macaroni　237
——— Orange flower　*ibid*
——— Palais

CONTENTS.

Biscuits   page

———— Palais royal   216
———— Punch   234
———— Queen   229
———— Royal maffapin   231
———— Savoy   228

CAKES.

———— Almond   133
———— Almond loaves   134
———— Bride   124
———— Bean   127
———— Beaned bread   136
———— Common   118
———— Cream   122
———— Crackling   146
———— Croqnante de fuelilletage   147
———— Clear   148
———— Feuelantine   146
———— Fashion   126
———— Flowers   132

Cakes

CONTENTS

Cakes   page
——— Gum   128
——— Homeycomb   129
——— Juices   130
——— Light   116
——— Lemon   129
——— Liquorice   132
——— Lisbon   139
——— Nuns   119
——— Orange flower   149
——— Pound   118
——— Puffs   138
——— Puis d'Amour   141
——— Do. small   144
——— Ratafia   120
——— Another way   230
——— Rice   126
——— Do.   127
——— Ratafia puffs   137
——— Savoy   121
——— Seed   *ibid*

CONTENTS,

Cakes   page

——— Saffron   123
——— Sugar paste   135
——— Sword knots   141
——— Snail   145
——— Violet   130
——— White with currants   117
——— Wormwood   131
——— Wafers, brown,   137

CONSERVES.

——— Dried   149
——— Chocolate   52
——— Coffee   *ibid*
——— Jonquill   *ibid*
——— Lemon   53
——— Lemon, white,   54
——— Orange flower   51
——— Orange   53

Conserve

CONTENTS

	page
Conserves	
——— Pomegranate	54
——— Saffron	51
——— Violet	50

CREAMS ICED.

Iced	186
——— Almond	191
——— Burgundy wine	188
——— Brown bread	95
——— Barley	200
——— Curd	187
——— Chocolate	192
——— Codling	197
——— Currant	198
——— Gooseberry	199
——— Hartshorn	189
——— Lemon	194
——— Lemon, White,	195
——— Orange	196

Cream

CONTENTS.

Cream	page
———— Pompadour	190
———— Pistachio	192
———— Do.	193
———— Preserve	198
———— Queens	187
———— Raspberry	193
———— Royal	96
———— Ratafia	196
———— Rhenish wine	187
———— Strawberry	186
———— Snow	189
———— Spanish	190
———— Do. another way	199
———— Steeple	201
———— Tea	69

CUSTARDS.

———— Baked	183
———— Almond	184

Cheesecakes

CONTENTS

	page
Cheesecakes	183
Caps, black,	208
——— Green	209

COMPOTES OR STEWED FRUITS.

——— Apples	68
——— Apricots	70
——— Do. green	71
——— Cherries	74
——— Lemon peels	69
——— Orange peels	ibid
——— Pears	70
——— Plumbs, green gages	72
——— Quinces	73

CANDIED OR PRALINED.

——— Almonds	38
——— Nuts	39

Candied

viii CONTENTS.

	page
Candied	
——— Do. Pistachio	40
——— Orange peel	41
——— Orange flower fresh	42
Candy, a method to make all sorts,	214
——— Caramel	216
Deserts, bills fare of,	211

FRITTERS.

——— Common	114
——— Apples	145
——— Almond	182
——— Curd	186
——— Clary	175
——— English	182
——— Italian	181
——— Orange	179
——— Olive	181
——— Plumb	177
——— Raspberry	*ibid*
——— Rice	178
——— Strawberry	177
——— Flummery hartshorn	204

Flummery

CONTENTS

	page
Flummery	
——— French	205
Fools raspberry	210
Ices with the juice of orange and lemon	75
——— For all sorts of liquid compositions	76
——— In moulds like fruit	78
——— Apricot	79
——— Barberry	85
——— Currants	80
——— Cedra	82
——— Grape	86
——— Jessamines	ibid
——— Muscadine	83
——— Orange flowers	86
——— Peach	80
——— Pear	81
——— Pine apple	84
——— Raspberry	81
——— Strawberry	ibid
——— Violets	86
——— With preserved fruits	87
——— With cream and fruits	88

Ices

CONTENTS

Ices   page
—— Apricots   92
—— Chocolate   89
—— Coffee   90
—— Do. white   91
—— Currants   92
—— Cherries   93
—— Pistachio nuts   88
—— Peach   93
—— Pine apple   ibid
—— Raspberry   92
—— Strawberry   91
—— With ripe fruits   94

JELLIES OF FRUIT.

—— Apple   110
—— Currants   104
—— Do.   105
—— Do. Black   109

Jelly

CONTENTS

	page
Jelly	
—— Gooseberry	108
—— Lemon	107
—— Orange	106

JAMS OF FRUITS.

—— Apricot	116
—— Cherries	115
—— Goosberries, green,	114
—— Raspberries, red,	112
—— ———, white,	113
—— Strawberries, red,	114
Jelly, Hartshorn,	203
—— Ribboned	202
Island floating	209

MARMALADES.

Marmalades	97
—— Apricot	ibid
—— Do.	98

Marmalade

CONTENTS.

Marmalade — page
——— Apples — 101
——— Orange — 99
——— Orange flower — 101
——— Peach — 102
——— Raspberry — 103
——— Strawberry — ib.d
——— Transparent — 100

PRESERVES.

Moist — 6
——— Apricots — 13
——— Do. green — ibid
——— Angelica — 14
——— Ananas or pine apples — 16
——— Barberries in bunches — 22
——— Drops — 23
——— Cherries, whole, — 11
——— Cherries, stoned, — 12
——— Cherries, double, — 18

Preserves

CONTENTS.

Preserves	page
——— Cucumbers	20
——— Currants	25
——— Figs	21
——— Goofberries, green,	17
——— Green gages	19
——— Grapes	21
——— Goofberries like hops	18
——— Lemons	6
——— Oranges	8
——— Pears	6
——— Peaches	10
——— Plumbs	24
——— Quinces	9
——— Rafpberries	25
——— Strawberries, whole,	24

Preferves

CONTENTS.

Preserves dry, of Fruits.

	page
—— Apricots	65
—— Barberries	64
—— Currants in bunches or sprigs	59
—— Cherries	55
—— Do.	56
—— Do. without sugar	*ibid*
—— Do. in bunches	57
—— Damsons	67
—— Figs, green	63
—— Gooseberries	58
—— Plumbs white	60
—— —— black	61
—— Green gage	66
Observations on preserving of fruits	1
Degrees of ripeness of fruits	11

PASTE

CONTENTS.

PASTE.

	page
—— Apricots	26
—— Do.	28
—— green	*ibid*
—— Apple	31
—— Lemon or Citron	*ibid*
—— Plumb	32
—— Peach	*ibid*
—— Quince	29
—— Red	30
Observations on fruit pastes	33
Paste, spun of apples, apricots, peaches and plumbs	*ibid*

PASTELS OR DROPS.

—— Barberries	48
—— Chocolate	44

Pastels

CONTENTS.

Paftels	page
—— Coffee	46
—— Currants	ibid
—— Lemon	43
—— Orange	47
—— Rafpberries	45
—— Ratafia of various forts	49

PASTE.

—— Orange flower	149
—— Puff	150
—— Do.	151
—— to fry or bake in	153
—— puff for fweetmeats	154
—— Queen	152
—— Royal	ibid
—— Rich	151
—— Rice	154
—— Spanifh	153

PIES.

CONTENTS.

PIES.

	page
—— Almond	163
—— Pear	157

Observations on Pickling.   241

—— Artichokes, young,	248
—— Barberries	249
—— Beet root	251
—— Cucumbers	241
—— —— in slices	242
—— Colliflower	248
—— Cabbage	247
—— Elder buds	250
—— Another in imitation of Indian bamboe	ibid
—— Grapes	246
—— Mushroom	245
—— Nasturtiums	252

Pickle

CONTENTS.

	page
Pickle	
—— Onions	246
—— Picalillo	251
—— Radish pods	249
—— Samphire	245
Vinegar to make, for pickles	240
—— Walnuts, black,	242
—— ——, white,	243
—— ——, green,	244
Sugars, to clarify	2
—— Its different degrees	3
—— For the liquid preserves	14
Sugar Plumbs, or Dragees,	217
—— Apples	225
—— Coriander	219
—— Cinnamon	220
—— Cardamum	221
—— Carraway feeds	222
—— Coffee	224

Dragees

CONTENTS.

	page
Dragees	
——— Chocolate	ibid
——— Violet	222
Syllabubs	205
——— Light	206
——— under the Cow	ibid
——— Snow	207

TARTS,

——— Almonds	166
——— Apricots	169
——— Angelica	171
——— Cream	162
——— Chocolate	165
——— Do.	166
——— Cowslip	167
——— Fashion	170
——— Goosberries, green,	171
——— Lemon	168

CONTENTS.

	page
Tarts	
—— Marmalade	156
—— Orange	198
—— Peach	160
—— Do.	161
—— Piſtachio	164
—— Do.	ibid
—— Plumb	170
—— Tarts	158
Trifle	202

WINES.

—— Britiſh	259
—— Birch	269
—— Cherry, Morella,	256
—— Currant	257
—— Another	270
—— Cowſlip	262
—— Canary	267

CONTENTS.

Wine	page
—— Damson	265
—— Elder	255
—— —— like claret	258
—— Fontiniac	261
—— Fine	ibid
—— Gooseberry	260
—— Grape	266
—— Lemon	256
—— Orange	253
Observations on wines	ibid
—— Quince	264
—— Raisin	254
—— Raspberry	268
—— Sage	262
—— Walnut	268

DIS-

CONTENTS.

DISTILLING.

	page
—— in general	1
—— in particular	5
Definition of spirits	6
—————— essences	7
—————— simple waters	8
—————— phlegms	9
—————— digestion	13
Of fruits and their different species	14
Of the aromatical and vulnerary plants	18
Of the various spices and seeds used in distillery	21
To make orange flower water	23
To make the neroly and orange flower water double	25
Receipt for the neroly	28
Of the orange flower water liquor	ibid
Receipt to make the same with neroly	30

Distilling

CONTENTS

Distilling	page
Of rose water	31
To have quintessence of roses	32
Of lilly water	34
To make lilly water liquor	ibid
A receipt for the common sort of liquor	35
A receipt for the double liquor	36
To make simple and double lilly water	ibid
To make the double water and quintessence	37
Of Carnation water	38
Another way	40
Jessamine water	41
Receipt for six quarts	42
A better way	ibid
Another way	ibid
Another way	43
Violet water	ibid
Jonquill water	45

January

January fruits in season.

Golden Pippins, Nonpareils, Pearmain-Apples, Medlars, dried Apples, Chesnuts, Royal Pears, St. Germain and winter Chaumontelle, Colmar, Rennets, and Russet Apples.

April fruits in season.

The same as in January, with Pomegranates, Winter Bonchretien, Pistachio Nuts, Almonds and Raisins.

June fruits in season.

All Sorts of Strawberries, Raspberries, Goosberries, Duke Cherries, Currants, Melons, the Masculine Apricots.

October fruits in season.

Peaches, Nectarines, Figs, Sweet Water Grapes, Green Gage Plumbs, St. Catharine Mulberries, Morella Cherries, Walnuts, Filberds, Arline Plumbs, Burgamot Pears, Buree Pears, Golden Pippins, Medlars, and Mulberries. I have mentioned only four months in the year, because fruit continues three months the same.

THE
FRENCH AND ENGLISH
GUIDE
TO ALL SORTS OF
CONFECTIONARY.

Proper Instructions for House-Keepers, to attain a more speedy, plain, and familiar Method of understanding the whole Art of Confectionary.

I T must be observed, that the first thing necessary, is perfectly to know the different degrees, or heights of clarifying or refining sugar, and agreeably to the fruit you have to preserve, in

order

CONFECTIONARY.

order to have them done in a higher degree of perfection, you must be attentive to make use of such degrees of sugar so refined, as is adapted to their different degrees of ripeness, as well as to their different sorts.

TO CLARIFY SUGAR.

IN proportion to three pounds of fine, lump, or powder sugar, which you are to put in a skillet or boiler; break into an earthen pan the white of an egg, with near a pint of fresh water, and beat them up all together with your hand to a white froth; then put the whole into the copper kettle, or pan, and set them on a clear and slow fire; when it begins to boil, do not fail to put a little more water in, and begin to skim it, till you see the scum is very white, and the sugar become pretty clear; that done, to clear it properly, sift it in a wet napkin, or silk sieve, and pass it thus into what vessel you please, till you want to make use of it.

FIRST

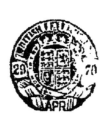

CONFECTIONARY.

FIRST DEGREE OF REFINING SUGAR.

The practitioner may take notice, that one pound of sugar is sufficient to make a trial of all the different degrees.

PUT the clarified sugar on a moderate but clear fire, to boil; you will know when it is to this first *degree*, by dipping one finger in it, and join it to another; by opening, if it draws to a small thread, and in breaking, returns to each finger in the nature of a drop, it is done.

Second degree, It is boiled a little more, and the thread extends further before it breaks, and is proved as the first.

Third degree, It is still boiled a little more, until it does not break, by extending the fingers half as much as is possible to do.

Fourth degree, It is boiled a little longer than the third; and is known to be the degree wanted, by not breaking, by all the extension that can be made with the fingers; and also when it forms in small pearls in the boiling, round and raised.

Fifth degree, It is known, by taking up some of the sugar with a skimmer, and dropping it into the boiling sugar again; if it forms a slanting streak on the surface.

Sixth degree, By a little more boiling, and tried in the same manner as the last.

Seventh degree, Which is known by dipping a skimmer into it; give it a shake, and blow through it directly; if it blows to small sparks of sugar, or kinds of small bladders, it is to the proposed qualification.

Eighth

Eighth degree comes with a little more boiling, which is known by the same trial; the difference only is, that the sparks or bladders are to be larger, and of a stronger substance.

Ninth degree, Is known by dipping a skimmer into it, and give it a turn over the hand; if it turns to large sparks, which clog together in the rising, it is done to this degree.

Tenth degree, Is done by a little more boiling, and proved by dipping two fingers in cold water, and directly into the sugar, and into cold water again; what sticks to your fingers, ought to roll up like a bit of paste, and to remain pretty pliant when cold.

Eleventh degree, Is proved by the last method, which, by a little more boiling, makes it harder.

Twelfth degree, Is known by the same method, as in the two last; the only difference is, that it ought to crumble between the fingers, being first dipped in cold water.

A Method for making all Sorts of moist Preserves.

SUGAR PEARS.

TAKE any quantity of pears, which should be but half ripe, make a split on their head cross ways with a knife, no deeper than the heart. After this is done, put a pan of water on the fire, and when it boils put your pears in it, and boil them in, with a slow fire, till they become a little soft; then take them off the fire, and throw them immediately in another pan of fresh water; have again another pan of fresh water, in which you squeeze three lemons, pare your pears and put them in that lemon water: they will turn as white as snow; then take a preserving

ing pan, put in it some of the first degree of your clarified sugar, put your pears in it, and let them boil about twelve minutes, taking care to take off all the scum they will throw; then take them out from the fire and put them in an earthen vessel; you will repeat this operation during four days running, and strain the sugar off every time, and boil it before you put the pears in, because, as you will perceive, the sugar always throws off a white scum, which must be taken off; and it is after that, you must put your pears in and boil them, as I said. When you see the syrup is very thick, and that your pears have well taken the sugar, put them in pots, and take care they should be well covered with syrup, or else they will soon turn mouldy. Cover them with paper or parchment.

PRESERVED LEMONS AND ORANGES.

TAKE any quantity of lemons, pare off the hard knobs of the rind, cut them into four quarters, or leave them whole, in piercing them by the ſtalk's end: have a pan of water on the fire, and throw your lemons or oranges in when it boils, and do them in, as much as you pleaſe, till you ſee you may get a pin by the head into them eaſily; then it is time to take them off, and put them in another pan of freſh water. When that is done, you clean them quarter by quarter from their kernels; and thoſe which are whole, muſt be cleaned alſo of all their pulp with a tea-ſpoon, taking care not to break them. As for what concerns the ſugaring of them, follow the ſame directions as above-mentioned for the pears.

MOIST QUINCES.

TAKE any quantity of quinces; cut them into four quarters; take well off the heart and the skin, and put them in a pan of water which you have on the fire; boil them thus till a skewer can get into them easily. Then take them off and put them upon a cloth to drain their water away; while this is doing, you set your preserving pan on the fire, with the quantity of sugar of the first degree which is necessary, and put your quinces in it; boil the whole well, till you see the sugar becomes very red. Then to know the proper time of its being done, take a little syrup with a spoon in a saucer, and let it cool; if it turns into a jelly, you must directly take away your quinces from the fire, and put them immediately quite hot into very dry pots, for should you let them be cold before you pot them, they would jelly, and you could no more make them fill all the

parts

parts of the pots without some air along with them. Take care that your syrup should always well cover your fruit, as I have said before.

MOIST PEACHES.

TAKE any quantity of peaches, rub well all their down with a cloth, and prick them with a large pin as much as you please. Have a pan of water on the fire, in which you put your peaches, and do them thus with a slow fire, taking a great care they should not boil, for you would run the risk of their bursting. When you perceive they are a little softened, take them off, and put them into fresh water; after which, you do for sugar just the same as we have said about the pears.

MOIST APRICOTS.

TAKE any quantity of apricots, make on the top of them a little opening with a small penknife,

knife, and by the stalk's end, thrust your knife in to push the stone out; try, at the same time, to do this so delicately, as not to squeeze it in your hand: then proceed, as before directed, for the peaches, with respect to what concerns the doing them in the pan over the fire; and, as before directed, for the pears, with respect to what concerns the sugar.

N. B. It is very proper to observe, that any fruit whatever, which is intended to be preserved, must be chosen rather green than too ripe; because when you blanch it in the water over the fire, it is apt to mash if too ripe, and gives a great deal of trouble; but when it is greener, it has more body to resist the boiling of the water.

WHOLE CHERRIES.

TAKE any quantity of cherries, cut half of their stalks, then put a preserving pan on the fire,

fire, with what quantity of clarified sugar you think proper, boil it well till you see your sugar at the sevehth degree, or *blowing height*; that is to say, you take a pierced spoon or strainer, you dip it into the sugar, and when you take it out blow through the holes; if your sugar sparkles and makes bladders, then it is time to put in your cherries; do it and skim them well, continuing so doing till your syrup is thick; or take the skimmer, dip it in the sugar, if it makes a sort of a *cobweb* in falling they are done enough: take them off and pot them, but do not fill the pots quite, for generally they ought to be filled deep with currant jelly.

STONED CHERRIES.

TAKE any quantity of cherries, pick out the stones with a little stick, have some clarified sugar in a sauce pan, put your cherries in and set them upon the fire till you see they begin to simmer;

mer, when you must directly take them off and pour them into an earthen vessel, there to remain till the next day, that they may discharge their juice. The next day you drain them from the sugar which you set on the fire to skim it well; after which you put your cherries in again, and proceed for the degree of doing as was said, for those which are preserved whole.

GREEN APRICOTS.

TAKE any quantity of apricots; have a pan of water on the fire, with about four shovelfuls of fine wood ashes in it, which you must boil well; after this you put in your apricots, you let them boil during three quarters of an hour in the lye, then take them out and throw them into fresh water, rubbing them well to take off the down which covers them; change them two or three times into fresh water, you will soon see your apricots

turn

turn of the finest green; take afterwards a small nail and pierce them *in the middle*, then put them in the first degree of sugar, and proceed as was said for pears.

N. B. It is proper to observe, that with respect to sugar in liquid preserves, the same directions are always to be followed; for when once you see your fruits have well taken the sugar, after having been passed four or five times in it, they all require the same degree of doing, unless you want to keep them a long while; in which case you may force them on the fire the value of two or three minutes longer than we have mentioned in speaking of the pears.

MOIST ANGELICA.

TAKE any quantity of angelica, it must be neither too green nor too ripe; to get it in its right point of maturity, as it is often later or sooner,

sooner, agreeably to the difference of the season in which you cut it; the gardeners are the proper people to apply to; they can tell you in what season it must be gathered. There are generally two different times of gathering it, the second is always the best, which are commonly about the month of August, because it has then lost its greatest strength. You cut it in small pipes and boil it in water as much as you please, after which, you put it in fresh water in order to take with a knife the skin, which comes off very easily, and leave but *the flesh* which is under the skin; you put it afterwards in the second degree of sugar, and proceed as for the other things as above-mentioned. You may if you please squeeze *six* lemons in your sugar at the moment you put your angelica in; as it is a fruit naturally dry, it will better connect the parts of the sugar together and prevent it from candying.

MOIST

MOIST ANANAS, OR PINE APPLES.

TAKE any quantity of ananas, cut them into four quarters, or in round slices, and pare off the skin, then take clarified sugar and water in equal quantities, put in the ananas and do them as the other above-mentioned fruits, taking care to skim them well during the time you are doing them; for it is very essential to remark, that when you are making any sort of preserves whatever, if you do not skim them well they are apt to grow sour, which occasions a great deal of trouble to repair them again. You must not boil the ananas in water first, as we have directed for the other fruits, because it would deprive it of its best substance and flavour.

GREEN

GREEN GOOSBERRIES.

TAKE any quantity of green goosberries, cut them with a pen-knife on one side, only to be able to get out the stones; throw them into cold water, and cover them with cabbage-leaves, then set them on a gentle slow fire; when they begin to boil, take them away from the fire, and let them grow cold in the same water till the next day, when you put them again upon hot ashes; as soon as they begin to get warm you will see them turn of a fine green, then take them off and throw them into cold water to make them firm; have clarified sugar of the first degree, put them in and proceed as usual, with this difference, only they must not boil long on the fire, for as it is a very delicate fruit, it would mash all away; therefore, better to avoid any risk of that sort, to give the sugar alone its degree of boiling, in keeping it well skimmed, than to do it when the goosberries are in.

GREEN HOPS.

TAKE any quantity of goosberries which you split with a pen-knife into four quarters, as far as the stalk's end only, taking care the quarters should not drop a part; then take a needle and thread, run them through of what length you please, and proceed afterwards precisely as we have directed for the whole goosberries.

DOUBLE CHERRIES.

TAKE any quantity of cherries from those which you have preserved with their stalks, and those without stones; open these last neatly, and introduce in them those with stalks, smoothing them well over, and place them in the stove with a gentle fire. This is what is called double cherries.

GREEN GAGES.

TAKE any quantity of green gages, prick them with a pin, put them in a pan with water, and set them on the fire; when you see the water is beginning to boil, take them off and leave them in that same water to cool till the next day, when you are to set them again on a very gentle fire, that they may turn green When you see they are green enough, you put them in a sieve to drain; then you take the first degree of clarified sugar, in which you add three parts water, then the plumbs, and set the whole on a slow fire to make them throw off their water; after which, you put them in a pan for two days, and then you add clarified sugar, and proceed as for the above preserves.

SUGAR PRESERVED CUCUMBERS.

TAKE any quantity of small cucumbers, prick them as much as you please with a needle, put them in a pan of water on a slow fire, and let them remain there till you see they are a little soft; then take them off and let them be in that same water till the next day, when you are to set them again upon hot ashes to green them. When that is done, throw them into cold water, then take some very light clarified sugar, to which you add three quarters water, put your cucumbers in and set the whole on the fire, that they may boil gently to throw off their water. Suppose that in doing this they should shrink, you may take them away and leave them for three or four days, then you will see they will have recovered; you may then continue to boil them gently on a slow fire, at three or four different times; after which you add sugar

gar to them and proceed quite the same as directed before for the other preserves.

SUGARED GRAPES.

TAKE any quantity of bunches of grapes which should not be quite ripe; make in every grape a small incision with a pen-knife to take the stones out, put them in a pan of water covered with cabbage leaves, and set them upon the fire, and proceed for the rest just as directed for the gooseberries, taking great care to keep the fire down and slow.

SUGARED FIGS.

TAKE some figs which should not be too ripe, prick them with a needle, put them in cold water, and set them on the fire till they become tender; then take them off and throw them into cold water; take the first degree of clarified sugar, put your figs in, and proceed as directed for the other preserves.

BARBERRIES IN BUNCHES.

TAKE any quantity of barberries without stripping them of their stalks, split them with a knife, take out all the seed which is in them, then tie them in little bunches; have clarified sugar which you set on the fire: when your sugar is at the ninth degree, put your little bunches in and boil them about ten minutes, after which you put them in a pan, and place them in the stove with a slow fire for three days running; at the end of which time, you take them from that sugar which you set again on the fire, to heighten it again to the above degree; for the barberries will have weakened it by throwing their juice in it. When that is done, put the bunches again in it, and place it as before in the stove for three whole days, after which you draw out your bunches from the sugar, and put them to drain on a wire grate, made on purpose for these sort of things; then you

you will range them on a horse-hair sieve, and replace them in the stove to dry them, and make what use you please of them.

BARBERRY DROPS.

TAKE any quantity of barberries, which you put in a pan without water, and set over the fire, stirring them continually with a spoon for fear they should burn. When you see they begin to sweat, that is to say, to throw their juice off, take a sieve, not too thick, and drain your fruit: when all the juice is well drained weigh it, and add two pounds of sugar, pounded and sifted very fine, to every pound of juice; put the whole together in a pan, and place it in the stove, after having well mixed it; and do not forget to stir it with a spoon three or four times in the day to melt well the sugar. When it has been three or four days in the stove, and you see it is come very thick, then you may dress it as you please, either in little cakes as big as a shiling, or pot it, or spread it upon tin plates, and replace them in the stove with a small fire, till it is of consistence enough to cut it with a knife, in what form you please.

ALL SORTS OF PLUMBS.

TAKE any sort of plumbs, prick them with a pin, that the water may penetrate in them; put them in a pan of water and set them on the fire till they are softened. You must take care they should be well blanched in the water; for if they were not well softened in the water, they are apt to shrivel and harden when you boil them in the sugar. When they are well softened in the boiling water, you change them into cold water, and do for the rest as we directed for the greengages.

WHOLE STRAWBERRIES.

TAKE any quantity of strawberries, pick off their stalks, and wash them well in cold water,

and

and drain them; take clarified sugar of the ninth degree and let it cool; when it is cold, put your strawberries in and set the whole again upon the fire, till they begin to feel the heat, take them off quickly and put them in a pan till the next day, when you put them again on the fire and boil them very gently, for fear they should mash; when the syrup is a little thickened take them off and pot them.

WHOLE RASBERRIES.

TAKE rasberries and do the same as we said about the strawberries.

WHOLE CURRANTS.

TAKE any quantity of currants, strip them of their stalks, pick off very carefully all those which happen to be squeezed, because these sticking themselves to those which are whole, that

spoils

spoils them; then proceed just the same as we have directed for the strawberries, except, you must not let them boil quite so long on the fire, being apt to burst; and, in order to give them a greater consistence, instead of leaving them only twenty four hours, as you do the strawberries in the sugar, you may leave the currants thus three days, because it is their nature to harden in sugar.

FRUIT PASTES.

PASTE APRICOTS.

TAKE any quantity of apricots very ripe, peel, stone, and cut them small, put them in a deep earthen pan, then take a large and deep kettle, fill it with water, and place in it the earthen pan in which the apricots are; boil them thus what is called *balneo maria*; when they have well boiled thus and thrown off their juice, take them off and pour them in a sieve to drain; when they

they are well drained, take a horse-hair sieve very shear or open, strain them well, after which you put them in a preserving pan on the fire to dry them a little; when you see they begin to make a thick paste, take them off, have a pair of scales, and weigh a pound and a half of very fine sifted sugar pounded in powder to every pound of fruit, put the whole again into the preserving pan, set it on the fire, keeping continually stirring with a spoon, till you see the sugar is well mixed with the apricots; take notice they must not boil, for then the sugar would melt too much; when that is done, put this paste in your tin moulds and place them upon tin plates in the stove: when they have got a good crust on the top, turn them to make them take one also at bottom; then after your paste is very firm, take a little knife and pass it all round the moulds to make them quit the paste, which you then put on a sieve in the stove, to make it crust by the sides; when the crust is well formed, take them off and put

them

them in boxes, or any thing elſe to keep them for uſe.

ANOTHER WAY.

PREPARE two pounds of ripe apricots as above; ſoak them pretty dry on the fire, and maſh them very fine; put a pound of ſugar, ſtir it well together on the fire, till the paſte quits the ſpoon; finiſh it directly in the moulds; and dry it rather hotter than the former paſte: it is done alſo, by putting as much weight of raw powder ſugar, when the fruit is ſoaked ſome time pretty dry, and ſtirring continually, till it is come to a good conſiſtence on the fire; finiſh as the laſt.

PASTE OF GREEN APRICOTS.

BEGIN by taking the down off, which is done by making a lye, with five or ſix handfuls of green wood-aſhes, ſifted and boiled, till the water

water is quite sleek, and smooth to the fingers; put in the apricots; let them soak, till the down comes off easily; stir the ashes pretty often, to hinder it from settling at bottom; take the pot off the fire, to clean the fruits one after another, and throw in fresh water as they are doing; then boil them in fresh water, tender enough to sift as usual; and boil the juice till it comes to a good consistence, stirring continually, for fear it should burn; weigh an equal quantity of fruit and sugar, and mix them very well together off the fire; put them in moulds directly, and dry as before.

QUINCE PASTE.

LET your quinces be full ripe, boil them till they are quite tender, drain and sift them as usual; reduce the marmalade (on the fire) to a paste-consistence, stirring continually, according to the quantity of quince-marmalade; refine a pound of sugar to three quarters of quinces;

mix

mix them together on a very flow fire without boiling, put it into what form you please directly, and dry as usual.

RED QUINCE PASTE.

TO make the paste of a fine red, bake the quinces in the oven a long while, then peel and sift them in a strong hair-sieve; dry the marmalade over a flow fire a little while, to about half the consistency of a paste; then to redden it the more, keep it a good while on a flow ashes-fire, stirring some time; and to add to this redness, put a little steeped cochineal, and reduce it on a flow fire, to a thick paste; that is, when it loosens from the pan; put as much sugar as marmalade, or paste, soak it a little while on the fire and let it cool, just enough to work it well with the hands, and finish directly as usual.

LEMON

CONFECTIONARY.

LEMON OR CITRON PASTE.

CUT off the hard knobs at both ends, core them through and through, boil them in water till they are tender; take them out and put them into cold water a moment, drain them by pressing them in a linen-cloth, to get the water out, then pound and sift them; upon a quarter of a pound of marmalade put half a pound of sugar, ninth degree, simmer it a while together, to mix, stirring continually, and finish as all others.

APPLE PASTE.

TAKE what quantity of golden pippins you think proper, which you boil whole in a pan of water without paring them; when you see they are well done, take them off and put them in a draining sieve; then take a horse-hair sieve very open, and strain them through; when that is done, put them in the preserving pan, and do just the same as we directed for the apricots.

PLUMB

PLUMB PASTE.

TAKE any sort of plumbs you please, put a pan of water on the fire; when it boils put your plumbs in, let them soak till you see they losen their skin; then take them off, strain them through a sieve, and put them in a pan over the fire, to make them throw off their water, keeping stirring them till you see your paste is a little thick; take them off, and continue as we said about the apricots.

PEACH PASTE.

TAKE any quantity of peaches, cut them small in an earthen pot, and do precisely as we directed you for the apricots.

CONFECTIONARY.

OBSERVATION ON FRUIT PASTES.

IT may be necessary to observe, that of all the different kinds of fruit pastes, heretofore mentioned, out of fruit season; marmalade of any sorts, mixed with sugar refined to the ninth degree, may be made use of; simmer it a little while together on the fire, and put it in moulds, in the same manner to dry in a very moderate heat; turn it over now and then, to dry equally of both sides. It also must be remarked, that pastes of any other kinds of fruits may be made by observing the quantity of sugar, according to the sharpness of the fruits.

SPUN PASTE.

TAKE either apples, peaches, apricots, or plumbs; put them in a pan of water on the fire, and do them as we directed before; then after you shall have strained them through a sieve, take cla-

rified

rified sugar, of the tenth degree; when done, take it off from the fire, and put your fruit in, which you boil as it were for a jelly: when you see your paste thickens, take it off, and spread it upon tin plates with a knife as thin as you can; put those tin plates in the stove for five or six days, with a slow fire; after that time your paste will be firm, then you take a knife and cut your paste as thin as you please; have little round sticks, cover them with that paste which you have cut, replace them again in the stove till the next day, then your paste will have taken the form of the sticks; take these off and keep them for use.

NUT BOMBOONS.

TAKE a pound of Spanish nuts, and boil them in an iron pan; when they are well boiled rub off their skin with a napkin, if some stick too

hard,

hard, pare it off with a knife; take a tin grater and grate your nuts very fine on a sheet of paper; then you take a pound of powdered sugar, to a pound of nuts, put it in a pan over a slow fire, when your sugar is all melted in stirring it perpetually with a wooden spoon, put your nuts in and work them well till all is well mixed, and pour it upon a tin plate; you have a wooden rolling-pin to spread it, which you must be very quick in doing, for it cools very fast; and when it is cold you cut it in what form you please; you must take care the sugar should not be too much melted, for it is very apt to soften when the nuts are joined to it.

LEMON OR ORANGE BOMBOONS.

TAKE a piece of loaf sugar, rasp the oranges or lemons with it, what of them sticks to the sugar you brush off upon a paper; then you pound in a mortar that same piece of sugar, and put it in a pan with that which is upon the paper, and which taftes of the lemon or orange; you fet it upon a gentle fire, in melting it flowly; after which you pour it upon a tin plate, which you muft before have rubbed with a little butter, or it will ftick to the plate; then you fpread it with the rolling-pin as you did for the nuts; (obferve the rolling-pin muft likewife be rubbed with butter, for fear it fhould ftick) when all that is done, and it is perfectly cold, then you cut it in what fhape you pleafe and fend it up.

BITTER ALMOND BOMBOONS.

TAKE bitter almonds, boil them in water to take off their fkin; after which you place them in the ftove to dry them well; when they are well dryed, take a grater and do as we directed for the nuts; you muft put the fame weight of fugar as almonds.

COFFEE

COFFEE-CREAM BOMBOONS.

TAKE about a pint of coffee made with water, put in it a pound of loaf sugar, set it on the fire, and boil it to the ninth degree, then you add a full pint of double cream, and let it boil again, keeping continually stirring till it comes to caramel height; to know when it is come to that point, you must have a bason of water by you, dip your finger in it, and put it quickly in your sugar, then in the water again to remove the sugar, which will have stuck to it; take a bit of it in your teeth, if it is hard in its crackling take it off, it is to the height required; pour it upon a tin plate, and proceed as we directed for the *lemon bomboons*. When it is warm you may cut it in little squares, or lozanges, or any other shapen *pastiles*, and draw a few strokes over them with a knife.

ORANGE-FLOWER BOMBOONS.

TAKE dryed, burnt, or what we call *pralined* orange flower, which you pound in a mortar, and pass through a sieve; then take half a pound of pounded loaf sugar, which you mix with your orange flower, and put in a pan over a slow fire, to melt it gently in stirring continually with a spoon; when it is all well melted, pour it on a tin plate, and do as we directed for the *lemon bomboons*.

CANDIED, OR RATHER PRALINED ALMONDS.

TAKE a pound of almonds, clean them well of their dust with a cloth, put them in a pan, with a pound of sugar and a little water, let them boil till they begin to sparkle, for this is a never failing mark of the right degree; then take them off the fire, and stir them well with

with a wooden spoon, till you see the sugar will turn gravelly, or gravel-like; then you set them again over a slow fire, to dissolve the sugar, keeping still stirring that the sugar may stick to the almonds; when you see your almonds come reddish, and are well covered with sugar, take them off, pour them in a sieve, cover them with a clean cloth, and put them in the stove, this makes them preserve their gloss.

PRALINED NUTS.

TAKE a pound of Spanish nuts without their shells, which you put in a pan with as much sugar, and do as we said for the almonds; you may give a little boiling to the almonds if you chuse to take off their skin, but then the sugar does not stick on them so well; observe, likewise, that you may, if you please, make all sorts of pralins * with clarified sugar, which you proportion in equal quantity, to the weight of fruit you want to pralin; your work will be certainly so much the finer, but generally they use loaf sugar.

PRALINED PISTACHIO NUTS.

TAKE a pound of pistachio nuts ready shelled, have a pan of water on the fire, when it boils put your nuts in it, let them boil thus a little, then take them off and rub off their skin; put them again in another pan with an equal quantity of sugar, and continue just as we directed you for the almonds.

---

* We beg leave to be allowed to use the words *praline*, and *to praline, pralined*, &c. which are quite French anglicised, as there is no English word to express the real idea of the French in this sort of preserving of almonds.

CONFECTIONARY.

PRALINED ORANGE PEEL.

TAKE any quantity of oranges, part them into four quarters, take their rind off, and take away very carefully all the white which is inwardly attached to it, so that there remain nothing but the very superficy of the yellow rind, cut it in strings as narrow as you please; when that is done, have a pan in which you put some clarified sugar, which you let boil a little, then put your orange rind in, let the whole boil together to the ninth degree; take it off and stir it with a wooden spoon, till you see your sugar is well mixed together: you may set it again on the fire if you chuse, keeping stirring till you see the sugar begins to dissolve, then take it off immediately; this will make your orange rind firm and cracking in the mouth.

As there are people who do not like the bitterness of the orange rind, you may, in such a

case,

case, give a little boiling to your rinds before you put them in sugar. Some other find that very bitterness an agreeable flavour in their mouth; then you must follow the above directions.

TO MAKE FRESH ORANGE FLOWER PRALINED.

TAKE any quantity of orange flowers, pick them carefully leaf by leaf; when that is done have a pan with what quantity of clarified sugar you need to have, boil it to the ninth degree then put your orange flower in; you will see that it will spoil all your sugar by the water it will throw off; let it boil thus till your sugar recovers as far as the first degree, then take it from the fire, and stir it till your sugar turn sand or gravel like; should it not dry so well as you would have it, set it again on the fire, and keep stirring it perpetually, till you see your sugar begins to melt; take it off immediately, and continue

tinue by stirring to reduce it into a sand: better to have a little more trouble in working your sugar to reduce it in sand, because then the orange flower does not take so much sugar, and has a better flavour; after it is dried you throw it in a sieve to drain the sugar from it, and keep nothing but the flower; then you place it in that sieve, in the stove, to finish drying it quite, stirring now and then for fear it should stick together; when it is well dried put it in your boxes and keep it for use.

LEMON DROPS OR RATHER PASTILS.

TAKE half a pound of pounded loaf sugar, sifted as fine as possible, put it in a plate, take three or four lemons which you squeeze over your sugar; mix it well with a spoon, till you see it makes what is called a *royal paste*, a little thickish, that you may take it upon a knife;

then

then take half a sheet of paper and cover it with little, round, and flat drops, which we call *pastils*, of the size of a farthing; place it in the stove with a slow fire till it is quite dry, and take it off from the paper; you may add to it, if you chuse, some of the skin of the lemon rasped or grated, but not chipped; for as it is a melting *pastil*, they would find some of the bits in their mouth, which is not quite so well.

CHOCOLATE PASTILS.

TAKE a little chocolate, which you put in a pan over the fire to melt it, stir it with a spoon; when it is well melted, take half a pound of loaf sugar, pounded in a mortar and sifted, which you dissolve in a little clear water. When that is done, put in your chocolate, if you find the paste too thick add a little water, enough to bring it to that degree of liquidity we specified for the lemons; then dress it on half

sheets

sheets of paper as we then directed, but do not put it in the stove for the heat softens chocolate; let it dry naturally in a cup-board, and when dry, take them off from the paper and put them in your boxes used for such kind of things.

RASPBERRY PASTILS.

TAKE half a pound of pounded loaf sugar on a plate, then a quantity of raspberries, which you squeeze through a sieve; when that is done, you add the juice to the sugar till it makes a paste of that consistency we specified in speaking of the lemons; dress it on the paper and put it in the stove till dry.

ANOTHER WAY TO MAKE RASPBERRY PASTILS.

MASH the raspberries, put in a little water, boil and strain them, then take half a pound of fine sugar, sifted through an hair sieve; just

wet

wet the sugar to make it as thick as a paste; put to it twenty drops of spirits of vitriol, set it over the fire, making it scalding hot, but not to boil: drop it on paper it will soon be dry; if it will not come off easily, wet the paper. Let them lie a day or two on the same paper.

CURRANT PASTILS.

DO exactly as we directed you for the raspberries; you have no occasion to put any water to these two sorts, because the juice of the fruit is enough of itself to dissolve the sugar, and make your paste as thick and as clear as you would have it.

COFFEE PASTILS.

TAKE half a pound of pounded loaf sugar, have about the quantity of two dishes of coffee made with water, which you put in your sugar, and mix well till you see it makes what is called

a royal

a *royal paste* a little thick, and proceed as before directed for the lemon drops.

You may, if you please, make them another way, *viz.* with ground coffee, which you sift very fine through a sieve, then adding a little water, as we said in speaking of the chocolate drops.

ORANGE PASTILS.

TAKE about a dozen oranges, squeeze out the juice, boil the rind very tender, cut out most of the white, and beat the yellow rind very fine; rub it through an hair sieve, and to a pound of the pulp put a pound and a half of fine sugar, sifted through an hair sieve; mix it well, and put in the juice till you make it thin enough to drop from a tea-spoon: drop it on glasses, and set it by the fire; let it stand there about two hours,

hours, and then put it in a stove; the next day turn it: it will be dry in twenty four hours.

BARBERRY PASTILS.

TAKE a good quantity of barberries, strip them off the stalks; put to them a little water, to keep them from burning; boil them, and mash them as they boil, till they are very dry; then rub them through an hair sieve, and afterwards strain them through a strainer, that there may be none of the black noses in it; make it scalding hot, and to half a pint of the pulp put a pound of the sifted sugar; let it scald, and drop it on boards or glasses; then put it in a stove, and turn it when it is candied.

RATAFIA PASTILS, EITHER OF APRICOT-KERNELS, OR HALF BITTER, AND HALF SWEET ALMONDS.

TAKE a pound of kernels or almonds, beat very fine with rose-water; take a pound of sifted sugar and the whites of five eggs beat to a froth, mix them well together, and set them on a slow fire; keep them stirring till they begin to be stiff; when they are quite cold, make them in little round drops: bake them after the long biscuit, on paper and tin-plates.

CONSERVES.

DRIED CONSERVES.

FOR all sorts of conserves, prepare the sugar after the ninth degree, according to the quantity wanted; they are all made much after the same manner: the only difference is in the quantity

tity of fruits propofed; few, who are not done with the fugar prepared to this degree, fhall be obferved: conferves are made with all forts of fweet-meats marmalade; ufe which you pleafe, fift it in a fieve, and foak it pretty dry over a flow fire, ufe about half a pound of the fugar prepared as fet forth, to a quarter of a pound of fweet-meats marmalade; take the fugar off the fire to work it well together; warm it a moment, and pour it in paper-cafes made for that purpofe; when it is cooled, cut it in cakes of what bignefs you pleafe.

VIOLET CONSERVE.

TAKE any quantity of violets, which you pick carefully leaf by leaf from their ftalk, put them in a little mortar and pound them well, take them out with a card and put them in a faucer; then take a little clarified fugar boil it to the ninth degree take it off from the fire, add your violets to it, and ftir it well with a fpoon, a spoon, till you see your sugar begins to thicken, pour it in a paper mould and let it cool; but before it is quite cold, mark with the point of a knife the different drops or *pastils* you intend to make of it, that you may afterward break them with more facility, and take them off from the paper.

ORANGE FLOWER WATER.

HALF a pound of clarified sugar being prepared to the ninth degree, take it off the fire, and pour a small spoonful of orange flower water in it; mix it well together, or any quantity to the same proportion; pour in the paper as the last.

SAFFRON CONSERVE.

THE sugar being prepared as before, have a little saffron powder soaked in water, and only pour a small quantity, just sufficient to colour the sugar of a pale saffron-colour.

JONQUILL CONSERVE.

DO exactly the same as we directed you for the violets; only take care when you work it with a spoon and the sugar is come to its proper point not to let it harden too much, for your conserve would not be so well melting in the mouth; it naturally dries enough upon the paper.

COFFEE CONSERVE.

TAKE a little coffee ground; have a pan with a little clarified sugar in; boil it to the tenth degree, take it off from the fire, and proceed just the same way as we directed for the other *conserves*.

THE *Chocolate Conserves*, are done in the same manner, with this difference only that yo must dissolve your chocolate in a small pan over the fire before you add the sugar to it; or if you do not chufe to diffolve it, grate it with a grater very fine it will anfwer the fame purpofe.

LEMON AND ORANGE CONSERVE.

TAKE a lemon or an orange, grate the rind with a tin grater, put the powder in a faucer, fqueeze the juice of the fruit over it, mix it well together with a fpoon, then boil fome fugar à tenth degree, becaufe what you put in it is a liquor, fince it is the juice and the grating of the fruit mixt together it lowers the fugar, which obliges to boil the fugar a little higher for this fort of conferve than for the others. When your fugar is boiled to the proper height you mix in it your compofition, and proceed on juft the fame for the reft as before directed for the the other conferves.

WHITE LEMON CONSERVE.

THIS is made differently as follows; boil a pound of the finest sugar to the eight degree; take it off the fire, and squeeze the juice of a lemon in it, at different times, stirring continually; it will whiten the sugar as white as milk, if properly done, take care not to drop any of the seeds in it; work it well together, and pour it in the moulds, when it is mixed of an equal substance, which you will prove by pouring some with a spoon, as any other jelly.

POMEGRANATE CONSERVE.

TAKE a good large ripe pomegranate of a fine colour; seed it one after another: then squeeze it in a linen-cloth, to ght the juice, which you boil, and reduce to half; put it to a pound of sugar, refined to the ninth degree; when it is half cold, work it well together, and dress it in the moulds as usual.

CONFECTIONARY.

To make dry preserves, or sweetmeats of all sorts of fruits.

TO DRY CHERRIES.

TAKE morella cherries, stone them, and to every pound of cherries, put a pound and a quarter of fine sugar, beat and sift it over your cherries, let them stand all night, take them out of your sugar, and to every pound of sugar put two spoonfuls of water, boil and scum it well, then put in your cherries, let your sugar boil over them, the next morning strain them, and to every pound of the syrup put half a pound more sugar, let it boil a little thicker, then put in your cherries, and let them boil gently, the next day strain them, and dry them in a stove, and turn them every day.

ANOTHER WAY

STONE a pound and a half of cherries, put them in a preserving pan, with a little water, when they are scalding hot, put them in a sieve, or on a cloth to dry, then put them in your pan again, beat and sift half a pound of double refined sugar, strew it betwixt every lay of cherries, when it is melted, set them on the fire, and make them scalding hot, let them stand till they are cold, do so twice more, then drain them from the syrup, and lay them separately to dry, dip them in cold water, and dry them with a cloth, set them to dry as before, and keep them in a dry place till you want to use them.

TO DRY CHERRIES WITHOUT SUGAR.

STONE the cherries, and set them on the fire, with only what liquor comes out of them;

let

let them boil up two or three times, shaking them as they boil; then put them in an earthen pot; the next day scald them, and when they are cold lay them on sieves, and dry them in an oven not too hot. Twice heating an oven will dry any sort of cherries.

TO DRY CHERRIES IN BUNCHES.

TAKE Kentish or morella, cherries, and tye them in bunches with a thread, about a dozen in a bunch; and when you have dried your cherries, put the syrup that comes out of them to your bunches; let them just boil, cover them close, the next day scald them; and when they are cold, lay them in sieves in a cool oven; turn them, and heat the oven every day till they are dry.

TO DRY GOOSBERRIES.

TAKE the large white goosberries before they are very ripe, but at full growth, stone and wash them, and to a pound of goosberries put a pound and a half of sugar, beat very fine, and half a pint of water; set them on the fire; when the sugar is melted, let them boil, but not too fast; take them off once or twice, that they may not break; when they begin to look clear, they are enough: let them stand all night in the pan they are boiled in, with a paper laid close to them; the next day scald them very well, and let them stand a day or two; then lay them on plates, sift them with sugar very well, and put them in the stove, turning them every day till they are dry; the third time of turning, you may lay them on a sieve, if you please; when they are pretty dry, place them in a box, with paper betwixt every row.

CONFECTIONARY.

TO DRY CURRANTS IN BUN-CHES OR LOOSE SPRIGS.

WHEN your currants are stoned and tied up in bunches, take to a pound of currants a pound and half of sugar; to a pound of sugar put half a pint of water; boil your syrup very well, and lay the currants into the syrup; set them on the fire, let them just boil, take them off, and cover them close with a paper; let them stand till the next day, and then make them scalding hot; let them stand two or three days with the paper close to them; then lay them on earthen plates, and sift them well with sugar; put them into a stove; the next day lay them on sieves, but not turn them till that side dries, then turn them and sift the other side: when they are dry lay them between papers.

TO DRY AMBER, OR ANY WHITE PLUMBS,

SLIT your plumbs in the seam; then make a thin syrup. If you have any apricot-syrup left, after your apricots are dried, put a pint of syrup to two quarts of water; if you have none, clarify single refined loaf sugar, and make a thin syrup. make the syrup scalding hot, and put in the plumbs; there must be as much syrup as will more than cover the plumbs; they must be kept under the syrup, or they will turn red: keep them in a scald till they are tender, but not too soft; then have ready a thick syrup of the same sugar, clarified and cold, as much as will cover the plumbs; let them boil, but not too fast, till they are very tender and clear, setting them sometimes off the fire; then lay a paper close to them, and set them by till the next day; then boil them again till the syrup is very thick; let them lie in the syrup four or five days, then lay them on sieves to dry: You may put some in codling jelly, first boiling the jelly with the weight in sugar, and put in the plumbs hot to the jelly. Put them in pots or glasses.

TO DRY BLACK PEAR-PLUMBS OR MUSCLES, OR THE GREAT MOGULS.

STONE your plumbs, and put them in a large earthen pot; make a syrup with a pound of single refined sugar and three pints of water; or if you have the syrup the white plumbs are dried out of, thin it with water, it will do as well as sugar; boil your syrup well, and when it is cold enough to hold your hand in it, put it to the plumbs; cover them close and let them stand all night; heat the syrup two or three times, but never too hot; when they are tender lay them on sieves, with the slit downwards to dry; put them in the oven, made no hotter than it is after bread

and

and pies come out of it; let them ſtand all night therein; then open them and turn them, and ſet them in a cool oven again, or in an hot ſtove, for a day or two; but if they are too dry, they will not be ſmooth; then make a jam to fill them with. Take ten pound of plumbs, the ſame ſort of your ſkins, cut them off the ſtones, put to them three pound of powdered ſugar; boil them on a ſlow fire, keeping them ſtirring till it is ſo ſtiff, that it will lie in a heap in the pan; it will be boiling at leaſt four or five hours; lay it on earthen plates; when it is cold, break it with your hands, and fill your ſkins; then waſh every plumb, and wipe all the clam off with a cloth: As you waſh them, lay them on a ſieve; put them in the oven, make your oven as hot as for your ſkins; let them ſtand all night, and they will be blue in the morning. The great white mogul makes a fine black plumb; ſtone them, and put them in the ſyrup with or after the black plumb; and heat the ſyrup every day, till they

are

are of a dark colour; they will blue as well as the muscles, and better than the black pear plumbs. If any of these blumbs grow rusty in the winter, put them into boiling hot water; let them lie no longer than to be well washed: Lay them on a sieve, not singly, but one on the other, and they will blue the better: put them in a cool oven all night, they will be as blue and fresh as at first.

TO DRY GREEN FIGS.

TAKE the white figs at the full bigness, before they turn colour; slit them at the bottom; put your figs in scalding water; keep them in a scald, (but not boil them) till they turn yellow; then let them stand till they are cold; they must be close covered, and something on them to keep them under water; set them on the fire again, and when they are ready to boil, put to them a little verdigrease and vinegar, and keep them in a scald till they are green; then put them

in

in boiling water; let them boil till they are very tender; drain them well from the water, and to every pound clarify a pound and half of single refined sugar, and when the sugar is cold put in the figs; let them lie all night in the cold syrup; the next day boil them till they are very clear, and the syrup thick, and scald them every day for a week; then lay them to dry in a stove, turning them every day; weigh your figs when they are raw; and when you clarify your sugar, put half a pint of water to a pound of sugar. If your figs grow too dry, you may put them in their syrup again; they will look fresh to the end of the year.

TO DRY BARBERRIES.

TAKE barberries, stone them, and tye them in bunches, or loose in sprigs, which you please; weigh them, and to every pound of barberries clarify two pound of sugar; make your syrup with something more than half a pint of water to a pound a pound of sugar; put the barberries into the syrup when it is scalding hot; set it on the fire, and let them just boil; then set them by, with a paper close to them; the next day make them scalding hot, doing so for two days; but be sure they never boil after the first time; when they are cold, lay them out on earthen plates; sift them well with sugar, and the next day turn them on a sieve; sift them again, and turn them every day till they are dry: Your stove must not be too hot.

TO DRY APRICOTS.

TAKE four dozen and a half of the largest apricots, stone them and pare them; cover them all over with four pound of sugar finely beaten; put some of the sugar on them as you pare them, the rest after: Let them lie four or five hours, till the sugar is almost melted; then set them on a slow fire till quite melted; then boil them but not too fast. As they grow tender, take them out

out on an earthen plate till the rest are done; then put in those that you laid out first, and let them have a boil together: put a paper close to them, and let them stand a day or two; then make them very hot, but not boil; put the paper on them as before, and let them stand two days, then lay them on earthen plates in a stove, with as little syrup on them as you can; turn them every day till they are dry, and scrape off the syrup as you turn them; lay them between paper, and let them not be too dry before you lay them up.

TO DRY GREEN GAGE PLUMBS.

MAKE a thin syrup of half a pound of single refined sugar, skim it well, slit a pound of plumbs down the seam, and put them in the syrup, keep them scalding hot till they are tender, they must be well covered with syrup, or they will lose their colour; let them stand all night,

night, then make a rich syrup, to a pound of double refined sugar, put two spoonfuls of water, skim it well, and boil it almost to a candy, when it is cold, drain your plumbs out of the first syrup, and put them in the thick syrup, be sure let the syrup cover them, set them on the fire to scald till they look clear, then put them in a china bowl; when they have stood a week, take them out, and lay them on china dishes, dry them in a stove, turn them once a day till they are dry.—If you would have them green, scald them with vine leaves, the same way as the green gages are done.

TO DRY DAMSONS.

GET you damsons when they are full ripe, spread them on a coarse cloth, set them in a very cool oven, let them stand a day or two, if they are not as dry as a fresh prune, put them in another cool oven for a day or two longer, till they are pretty dry, then take them out, and lay them in a dry place; they will eat like fresh plumbs in the winter.

To make all Sorts of stewed Fruits, or rather Compotes.

COMPOTES OF APPLES.

TAKE any sort of apples, cut them in halves, take off the core and pare them very neatly, and in proportion as you cut and pare them throw them in a bason of water, for fear they should blacken; have a pan on the fire with clarified sugar in, very light, that is to say, half sugar and half water; let it boil that you may skim it a little, then put your apples in and do them gently, taking care your sugar should not boil too fast, because in such a case they would wash all to a pulp. When you see that your apples are well done, take them off from

the

the fire, and let them cool in the sugar; for should they be too much done, in cooling in the sugar itself, they grow firm again, so set them in your ashes; but, if you should perceive your syrup is too thin, you may, after you have taken off your apples, set it again over the fire, and give it what degree or *height* you please.

COMPOTES OF ORANGE OR LEMON PEELS, COMMONLY CALLED, RAILLADINS.

TAKE the rind of either lemons or oranges, cut in four quarters; take off all the white of the inside, and keep but the superficy of the peel, or the outward rind; cut them in long threads as fine as you can, put them in a pan of water over the fire, boil them well, till in taking a bit between your fingers you may squeeze it to nothing; then take them off and change them into cold water; have another pan with very light clarified sugar in, put your *railladins* in and let them boil well, till you see they have well taken the sugar, take them off and put them in your glasses.

COMPOTES OF PEARS.

TAKE pears, which should not be too ripe, split them by the head's end with a knife, put them into a pan of water, and boil them till they are a little softened, take them off and change them into cold water: have another little pan of fresh water in which you squeeze two lemons, after which pare your pears neatly, and put them in that lemon water to whiten them: take then another pan with clarified sugar very light, and put your pears in till you see they have well taken the sugar, and they are well done.

COMPOTES OF APRICOTS.

TAKE any quantity of apricots, split them on one side to take out the stone, put them in a pan of water, and set them over the fire, boil them

them very gently for fear they should mash; when you see they are well softened, take them off and change them into cold water; take clarified sugar, put your apricots in, give them a little boiling, then take them off and set them in your china dishes.

COMPOTES OF GREEN APRICOTS.

TAKE any quantity of green apricots, then two handfuls of salt, which you wet with a little vinegar; take a coarse towel, put your apricots in it along with the salt, and rub them well in the towel till you see the apricots have lost all their down; be careful not to do them so hard as to break their skin; when that is well done, throw them into fresh water to make them lose the salt and vinegar, which is done by giving them three or four different successive fresh waterings; when you see your apricots are well cleaned, prick them well with a pin, set them in a pan of water on the fire, and boil them as much as you

please;

please; when they are sufficiently done, take them off from the fire, and let them cool in that same water till the next day, when you are to set them again on the fire in that same water, and as soon as it begins to boil take them off and change them into cold water; then take another pan with clarified sugar of the first degree, put your apricots in, let them simmer on a slow fire till you see they begin to turn very green; you must not let them be quite done the first time you put them in sugar, they must have then but one bubble in that degree of sugar, then take them off and let them stand till the next day, when they shall have thrown off all their water, and turn of the most beautiful green.

COMPOTES OF GREEN GAGES.

TAKE green gages, which you prick with a pin, and set on the fire in a pan of cold water, till you see they are a little softened; then take them

them off and let them cool in the same water, when that is done you take clarified sugar of the tenth degree, put your plumbs in it, and set them again on a very slow fire to make them throw off their water and turn green; you must also cover your pan during this second operation with a tin-plate, that they may not lose their steam, which makes them greener; after which you take them off and dress them in your china dishes.

COMPOTES OF QUINCES.

TAKE quinces, which you cut into four quarters, and take of their cores and pare them; set them in a pan of water on the fire, boil them as much as you please; when you find them done enough take them off from the water, and put them on a cloth to drain; then take another pan with clarified sugar of the first degree, and put your quinces in and let them do gently upon a slow fire that they may be very mellow: If you

you would have them red, you have but to cover them as foon as you putt hem on the fire with a tin plate, and leave it on till they are quite done; then take them off and drefs them in your china difhes. If you fee your fugar is in jelly, you muft put them directly in your china difhes and pour your fugar over them.

COMPOTES OF CHERRIES.

TAKE cherries, and cut off half of their ftalks; have clarified fugar, put your cherries in, and let them boil till you fee they are done enough; then take them off foom the fire, and let them ftand till they are grown cold enough to take them all one by one, and fet them on their ftalk upwards in your china difhes; and pour your fugar over them.

A method to make Fruit Ices.

ORANGE AND LEMON ICES.

TAKE clarified sugar in a pan of the ninth degree, then take three lemons or oranges, pare very neat the outer rind without any of the white which is under it, and drop it in the sugar, where it must remain about one hour to let it take well the taste of it. When that is done take the same three oranges, or lemon which you have pared, cut them by the middle, and squeeze well their juice in your sugar; then pass the whole through a sieve into another pan, and put this composition mixture from this last pan into the iceing pot, which we call *sabottere*. You may add if you please, the juice of three or four lemons to your *orange ice*; it will fatten the sugar and make your ices more mellow.

THE WAY TO ICE ALL SORTS OF LIQUID COMPOSITIONS.

WHEN your composition is put in the *sabotiere*; take some natural ice and put it in a mortar, when it is reduced into a powder strew over it two or three handfuls of salt; then take your pails, put some pounded ice in the bottom, and place your *sabotiere* in those pails which you fill up after with ice to bury the *sabotiere* in. You must take care in the beginning to open your *sabotiere* in order not to let the sides freeze first, and on the contrary detach with a pewter spoon, all the flakes which stick to the sides, in order to make it congeal equally all over in the pot. Then you must work them well as much as you are able, for they are so much the more mellow as they are well worked; and their delicacy depends entirely upon that. You must not wait till they are thoroughly iced to begin to work them, because

because they would become too hard and it is not possible to dissolve what is congealed in lumps or pieces. When you see they are well congealed you let them rest, taking care for this time there should be some which stick to the sides of the icing-pot: this will prevent them from melting and make them keep longer in a right degree of icing.

N. B. Suppose your composition should not congeal so quickly as you could wish through the melting of your pounded ice, you may change that ice in the same manner as you put it before; for as there is always a hole at the bottom of those buckets, you may let the water of your melted ice run off, by taking out the stopper without disturbing the *sabotiere*, then fill your buckets up again as you did before continuing rolling your *sabotiere* till you see your composition is congealed to the point you wish.

THE

THE WAY TO MOULD ICES IN ALL SORTS OF FRUITS.

WHEN your compofition is perfectly congealed, take a fpoon and the moulds you want to make ufe of; fill thefe well with your ices as quickly and dexteroufly as you can: you muft have befides juft ready by you a bucket with pounded natural ice, and a great deal of falt; there you put your moulds in proportion as you fill them, and cover them directly with pounded ice and falt, continuing fo doing to every mould you fill up till you have filled them all. When that is done you cover them quite and fet them a full hour in that ice. When you want to take off what is in your moulds, you take a pan of water, and firft wafh well thofe moulds one after the other to rub off all the falt which fticks round them, then you open your moulds put their contents in a china difh and fend them up. You may give to
every

every one of your ices the very colour of the fruit they represent; but then you must have your colour ready by you, and with a very fine pencil point them quickly, in which case they must likewise be served directly, or at least you must put them in the *cave*; then your *cave* must have been set in a bucket and prepared half an hour before you take your fruits from their moulds: in that *cave* you are then to set them after they are coloured, till the moment comes of serving them; your fruit is certainly finer and takes the downy look of the natural one.

APRICOT ICE.

TAKE very ripe apricots, cut them very small in a sieve, which you place over a pan, squeeze them well with a spoon through that sieve, and after it is done, add some clarified sugar to it, take afterwards about twenty almonds from the stones of those very apricots, pound

pound them very fine in a mortar, moistening them with a little clear water; when they are well pounded mix them with your apricots; if you see your mixture is too thick, you squeeze in the juice of three or four lemons and a little water, till you see it is neither too clear nor too thick, then put it in the *sabotieres*, and proceed as before directed.

PEACH ICES.

TAKE very ripe peaches, skin them neatly, cut them in small bits, and continue just the same as we directed you before for the apricots.

CURRANT ICES.

TAKE currants picked from their stalks and squeeze them through a sieve, then take clarified sugar, boil it to the ninth degree, add it to your currant's juice, squeeze four lemons besides in it if you chuse, it will render them but the more

CONFECTIONARY.

more mellow, strain them through a sieve a second time, and put them in the *sabotieres* to make them congeal, as we said for the lemons, to which I refer for the rest of the proceedings.

RASPBERRY ICES.

TAKE raspberries, which you squeeze through a sieve, and proceed as before directed for the currant ices.

STRAWBERRY ICES.

DO as we directed for the currant ices.

PEAR ICES.

TAKE pears, cut them in halves in a pan of water, which you set on the fire and boil as it were for stewing or *compotes*. When you see they are well done take the cores and the skin off, cut them very small in a pan, add some clarified

sugar

sugar of the first degree to them, and a little water, give the whole together another boiling, till it is well reduced into a pulp; then take them off from the fire and put them in a sieve, through which you squeeze them well; when that is done, if your pulp is too thick, add the juice of four lemons, some water, and a little more sugar, if they should not be sweet enough; then pass them a second time through the sieve, and put them in the *sabotiere* to make them congeal, in following our directions as above.

CEDRA ICES.

TAKE a piece of loaf sugar, you have a fresh and sound cedra, which you rasp or grate over a paper on that piece of sugar, scraping with a knife what sticks upon the sugar of the skin of the cedra; when you have thus taken off all the superficy or outer rind of your cedra, by rasping or grating it on the sugar, you take a little clarified

sugar

sugar boiled to the ninth degree, which you add to the raspings or gratings of the cedra, with what quantity of juice of lemons you think requisite for the quantity of ices you are willing to make, and a little water; pass the whole through a sieve and put it in the *sabotiere* to congeal as we said before.

N. B. You may likewise make cedra ices with preserved cedra, which, in that case, you are to pound in a mortar, and boil it in a very light sugar, then proceed afterwards just as we directed for the other cedra.

MUSCADINE ICES.

TAKE one ounce of elder flower, which you put in a *sabotiere*, pour upon it about half a pint of boiling water, cover your sabotiere with its lid, thus let it draw about half an hour, make then a composition precisely, as it were to make a plain a plain lemon ice, and as directed in that article; to that compofition add your infufion of elder flower, pafs the whole through a fieve, and put it in the fabotiere to congeal as we have explained.

N. B. You may make this fort of ice with white currants when it is the feafon, proceeding as it were to make a plain currant ice, and adding to it afterwards your infufion of elder flower, &c.

ANANA, OR PINE APPLE ICE.

TAKE any quantity of ananas, take the fuperficy off their fkin, cut them fmall, and pound them in a mortar; when they are well pounded you muft fqueeze them in a cloth to get all the juice; you muft pound them feveral times, becaufe, as in pounding them, you draw nothing more than their juice, and you cannot make them foft and liquid enough to make them all pafs

through

through the cloth, which obliges you to put them several times to the mortar; when that is quite done as it should be, you sqeeze in it the juice of four lemons, or more if you chuse, you put your clarified sugar to it boiled to the second degree: if you see then that your composition is too thick, you may add a little water to it, then pass the whole through a sieve to make them congeal, as we said before.

BARBERRY ICES.

TAKE barberries, which you put in a pan without water, set it over a very gentle fire, stirring them continually; when they are warm you take them off and pass them through a sieve in a pan, add sugar of the second degree to that liquor, and if it proves too thick you may put some water to it, but no lemon juice by any means, for the barberries are already acid enough of themselves, without increasing that acid with the addition

addition of the lemon; therefore put your compofition as above in your *fabotiere*, to congeal according to our former directions.

GRAPE ICES.

TAKE ripe grapes picked from their ftalks, pafs them through a fieve, mix your fugar with the juice of four lemons fqueezed in it; pafs the whole together a fecond time through a fieve, and put it afterwards in the *fabotiere* to congeal according to our former directions.

ICES OF VIOLETS, JESSAMINES, AND ORANGE FLOWERS.

POUND a handful of violets, and pour about a pint of hot water upon; let them infufe about an hour; put half a pound of fugar; when it is properly diffolved, fift through a napkin. The jeffamine is done after the fame manner, to make the liquid tafte more of the different

flowers,

flowers; pour it several times from one pan into another before sifting; the same with the orange flowers; those different infusions are also mixed with cream, instead of water.

DIRECTIONS FOR THE ICES MADE WITH PRESERVED FRUITS.

THERE are none of the ices which we have directed you how to make with fresh gathered fruit, but may be made also with that same sort of fruit after it has been preserved; in which case you are to proceed thus:

Take your preserve of whatever sort it is, put it in a bason, mash it well and dissolve it as much as possible with a spoon, some lemon juice and a little water to bring it to a pulp; pass it through a sieve: should they not be sweet enough add as much clarified sugar as is required, and when you have passed them through your sieve, put them in your *sabotiere*, and make them congeal by working them as we directed before.

A Method for making Cream Ices.

PISTACHIO NUTS CREAM ICES.

TAKE any quantity of cream in a pan, put in another four yolks of eggs for every pint of cream you are to employ; pound your pistachio nuts very fine in a mortar, and put them in the pan where you dropped your yolks of eggs; mix the whole together, add some pounded loaf sugar to it, keeping stirring continually, then add your cream by little and little, in stirring and turning till the whole is mixed properly together; then set your pan over the fire, and keep stirring with a wooden spoon till you see your composition is willing to boil, when you are to take it off immediately; for from the moment you set your composition over the fire till that it offers to boil,

it

it has a sufficient time to incorporate well and thicken sufficiently, without need of boiling; and should you let it boil, you would run the risk to make your cream turn into whey, on account of the yolks of eggs, which would do too much. Take great care likewise your cream should be very fresh and sweet, for, otherwise, as soon as it would feel the warmth it would all turn into curds and whey; therefore, for all these considerations, you are to take care to stir it well and continually, from the moment you set it on the fire to that you take it off; after which you pour it into a sieve to pass it in a pan, then put it in the *sabotiere* to make it congeal after the usual manner.

CHOCOLATE CREAM ICES.

TAKE any quantity of chocolate, melt it over the fire in a small pan; when melted, you pour it into that where you are to make your cream;

cream; you break your yolks of eggs in it, and continue to proceed as directed to make the piſtachio-nuts cream, for there is no other difference but that of the chocolate in the ſtead of the piſtachios; and, as for the reſt of proceeding, you are to follow the ſame directions as in piſtachio-nuts cream.

COFFEE CREAM ICES.

TAKE about a pint of coffee made with water, and rather ſtrong, when ſettled draw it clear, and add half a pound of ſugar, ſet it on the fire, and let it boil till your ſugar is to the ninth degree; take it off from the fire and let it cool, after which you make your cream as we ſaid, with the yolks of eggs, and put your coffee in, then for boiling, fiefting, and icing, proceed as uſual.

WHITE

WHITE COFFEE CREAM ICES.

PREPARE your cream as we have explained, take then a quarter of a pound of coffee in grain, which you roast as it were to make coffee with water; when roasted put it in a fine cloth, which you tye as a bag, and throw it quite hot in your cream; then set it on the fire keeping stirring till it offers to boil; take it off, pass it in a sieve, &c. &c. and proceed as usual for the rest.

STRAWBERRY CREAM ICES.

TAKE any quantity of strawberries, squeeze them through a sieve; when done, you mix your cream and your sugar, boil it, and repass the whole through the sieve again, then proceed as usual.

APRICOT

APRICOT CREAM ICES.

TAKE any quantity of apricots, squeeze them through a sieve, join what quantity of cream and sugar you want to make, and proceed as for the strawberries.

RASPBERRY CREAM ICES.

TAKE your raspberries, squeeze them through a sieve, add what cream and sugar you think to have need off, and proceed as for the rest as for the strawberres.

CURRANT CREAM ICES.

TAKE currants ready picked from their stalks, squeeze them through a sieve, add your cream and sugar, and proceed as directed for the strawberries.

PEACH

PEACH CREAM ICES.

TAKE any quantity of peaches, peel them, squeeze them through a sieve, add your cream and sugar, and proceed as for the strawberry cream ices.

ANANA OR PINE APPLE CREAM ICES.

TAKE any quantity of ananas, do as we directed you for the ices of ananas; when it is so far ready, only add your cream to it, and pass the whole through a sieve, and put it in the *sabotiere* to congeal as usual.

CHERRY CREAM ICES.

TAKE any quantity of cherries, take out their stones, squeeze them through a sieve, join what cream and sugar you think to have need off, and proceed as usual.

OBSERVATIONS ON ICES, MADE WITH RIPE FRUITS.

THE ices which we have juft given you directions for, viz. *Strawberry, Apricot, Rafpberry, Currants, Peach, Anana,* and *Cherry-Cream-Ices,* muft firft be made as it were for making them with the fruit alone; when they are fo far prepared, you join your cream cold to them fuch as you buy it, for fhould you put it warm, as generally moft of thefe fruits are acid, you would run the rifk of making your cream turn directly into curds and whey; therefore you are to put your cream cold to your fruit; and if you want to have your ices very mellow, you muft make ufe of the double cream which is thicker.—You may alfo make all thofe forts of ices with the preferved fruit of eace kind as we faid in the directions, for the ices made with preferved fruits, by putting your *preferves* in a bafon, and mafhing them

them well with a spoon, and the juice of four lemons and then the cream instead of water; for it is usual always to add some water to your fruit besides the lemon juice, in order to render them more fluid; now in the stead of that little water you put your cream to any quantity you please without bounds.

BROWN BREAD CREAM ICES.

TAKE any quantity of cream, prepare it as we said befor, boiling it alone with yolks of eggs and the sugar, pass it through a sieve and put it in the *sabotiere*; when your cream begins to congeal, have crumbs of brown bread, which you have grated and sifted as fine as powder, put it in the *sabotiere* and continue to work your cream for congealing.——You may also make this sort of cream with plain cream alone, without yolks of eggs, nor boiling, adding only a proper quantity of powdered loaf sugar, and set it to congeal,

congeal, and when it begins to ice, then put your fifted crumbs of brown bread. But take care to have it so finely sifted, for it renders it infinitely more agreeable to the mouth. As for icing see the receipt in page 76, the way to ice all sorts of liquid compositions.

ROYAL CREAM ICES.

TAKE any quantity of cream, join to it yolks of eggs in proper proportion as we said in the pistachio nuts put a little half pounded coriander, cinnamon, orange, or lemon peel; add some pounded loaf sugar, and set it on the fire as we said before, till the moment you see it is going to boil; then pass it through the sieve and set it to ice as usual.

TEA CREAM ICES.

MAKE tea very strong in a tea-pot, have your cream ready mixt with the proper quantity of of sugar and yolks of eggs, pass your cream through a sieve, pass likewise your tea over it, mix the whole well with a spoon, when that is done put it in the *sabotiere* and make it congeal according to the usual method.

Directions for making Marmalades.

APRICOT MARMALADES.

TAKE any quantity of apricots, peel them well, cut them very small in a pan and weigh what you have; then take pounded and sifted loaf sugar, and weigh the same quantity of it as you have of apricots. Have a large pan where you put both your apricots and your sugar together, set them over the fire and stir them continually with a wooden spoon till they are quite done. The way to know when it is come to its right point is to have a card and put with your spoon a little of your marmalade upon it, then turn it upside down, if it falls off you must continue stirring,

stirring, for fear it should burn, for it is not done; repeat then the trial upon your card several times, and when it sticks and does not drop off from the card it is right, take it from the fire and pot it.

ANOTHER WAY.

TAKE any quantity of apricots, cut them very small in a pan without peeling; weigh in proportion three quarters of a pound of clarified sugar to every pound of apricots. Put that sugar alone on the fire and boil it to the twelfth degree or breaking height, then take it off and put your apricots in. Set your pan again on the fire, and boil them along with that sugar till they come to the point we specified above, trying the same experiment.

N. B. You may do this marmalade again differently if you want to make it still finer; which is to take your apricots rather less ripe; that is to say, a little hard; cut them small and boil them in a pan with a little water, keeping stirring till they are quite mashed into a pulp; then you take them off, pass them through a sieve and weigh them, add to every pound of fruit, three quarters of a pound of either clarified, or pounded and sifted loaf sugar, as we said before, then boil the whole together as we said in both our articles, and pot them for use.

ORANGE MARMALADE.

TAKE the clearest Seville oranges you can get, cut them in two, then take all the pulp and juice out into a bason, pick all the seeds and skins, boil the rinds in hard water till they are tender, (taking notice to change the water two or three times while they are boiling) then in a mortar add to it the juice and pulp, and put them in the preserving pan, with double the weight of loaf sugar, set it over a slow fire, boil it a little more than half an hour, then put in pots for use.

TRANSPARENT MARMALADE.

TAKE very pale Seville oranges, cut them in quarters, take out the pulp, and put it into a bason, pick the skins and seeds out, put the peels into a little salt and water, let them stand all night, then boil them in a good quantity of spring water till they are tender, then cut them in very thin slices, and put them to the pulp, to every pound of marmalade put a pound and half of double refined sugar, beat fine, boil them together for twenty minutes; if it is not clear and transparent, boil it five or six minutes longer, keep stirring it gently all the time, and take care you do not break the slices; when it is cold, put it in jelly or sweet-meat glasses: they are pretty for a desert of any kind.

MARMALADE OF APPLES, OR PEARS.

PEEL and cut any quantity of golden pippins in thin flices, boil them with a little water very tender, pafs them through a fine hair fieve and put the marmalade on the fire to reduce the liquid part; then put it to as much weight of the ninth degree of clarified fugar on a flow fire, to fimmer a little while, ftirring it continually, to mix them both well together, then put it in pots for ufe, obferving to let it be cold before you cover it, proceed for doing the pears in the fame manner.

ORANGE FLOWER MARMALADE.

AFTER your flowers are properly picked, fcald them near the fpace of a minute, then put them in water, that has had a little allum diffolved in it; boil fome other water, in which you squeeze near half of the juice of a small lemon, and boil the flower in it till they feel tender; then put them into fresh water again, with the same quantity of lemon juice, and drain them in a napkin to pound; and mix two pound of this marmalade with five pounds of sugar of the first degree, or any quantity in proportion; finish as usual.

PEACH MARMALADE.

TAKE any quantity of peaches, cut them small, put them in a pan with a little water, boil them till they are well mashed, keeping stirring continually; then you take them off and pass them through a sieve; when sifted, you weigh them and put them again in the pan, and boil them again till you see that the water they give is a little reduced; when so, weigh an equal quantity of sugar as you had of peaches, and put it by little and little into your pan, and continue as we directed you for the apricot marmalade.

You

You may chuse whether you use clarified or pounded loaf sugar, it is quite indifferent, then proceed with your peaches, just as we directed you for the apricots.

RASPBERRY MARMALADE.

TAKE any quantity of raspberries, pass them through a sieve, and continue precisely as we mentioned in the article of peach marmalade.

STRAWBERRY MARMALADE.

TAKE any quantity of strawberries, squeeze them through a sieve, and continue to proceed for the rest as we directed you in the article of peach marmalade.

Directions for making of Fruit Jellies.

IT is necessary to observe, that as these jellies are directed to be done much in the same manner as the marmalades; that a material difference must be observed in sifting the different sorts of fruits, not to force any thing but the juices, which make the jellies clearer, and ought, for that purpose, to be strained in linen cloth.

CURRANT JELLY.

TAKE any quantity of currants, pick them from their stalks, and put them in a pan over the fire, with a little water; boil them till you see they are all well bursted, then take them off and pour them in a sieve to drain; when they are well drained, you set that liquor again in a pan over the fire and boil it well, skim it till you see it gives no more scum, when you are to take it off and weigh it: then take three quarters of a pound of clarified sugar of the twelfth degree to every pound of liquor, which you will boil by itself; when it is comes to that degree, pour in your currant juice, boil the whole together, and

continue

continue skimming it well till it is come to its proper consistency for a jelly, which you try thus: Pass your skimmer through your liquor, and lifting it up let the liquor fall; if it falls clear, let it boil longer; if it makes a kind of a cobweb, and then little bullets in falling from the skimmer, take it off from the fire, it is done; pot it quite hot, for should you let it cool in the pan, it would jelly and would not look well in the pots afterwards.

ANOTHER METHOD OF MAKING CURRANT JELLY.

WEIGH seven pounds of red currants without being picked; boil with a glass of water, and sift in a sieve; weigh the gross substance that does not sift; if there remains half a pound, there ought to be near five pound of juice; put this juice in a pan, with as many pounds of pounded sugar, which you pour in it by little and little; or to keep it pretty tartish, put only five pounds;

pounds; boil, stirring continually; when it has boiled a moment, take it off the fire to skim it and boil a little while longer; let it rest in the pan, and skim it again very clean.

ORANGE JELLY.

TAKE half a pound of hartshorn shavings, and two quarts of spring water, let it boil till it be reduced to a quart, pour it clear off, let it stand till it is cold, then take half a pint of spring water, and the rinds of three oranges pared very thin, and the juice of six, let them stand all night, strain them through a fine hair sieve, melt the jelly, and pour the orange liquor to it, sweeten it to your taste with double refined sugar, put to it a blade or two of mace, four or five cloves, half a small nutmeg, and the rind of a lemon, beat the whites of five eggs to a froth, mix it very well with your jelly, set it over a clear fire, boil it three or four minutes, run it through your jelly bag several times till it is clear, and when you pour it in your bag take great care you do not shake it.

LEMON JELLY.

TAKE four lemons, grate the rinds very fine into a pint and half of spring water, let it lie an hour, and then put to it the whites of five eggs well beaten; half a pound of sugar, and the juice of four lemons; when the sugar is melted, strain it through a thin sieve or strainer; then take a little powder of turmeric, tied up in a piece of muslin, and lay it in a spoonful of water till it is wet; then squeeze a little into the jelly to make it lemon colour; but not too yellow: set it over the fire, skim it, and when you see it jelly, put it in glasses; if it boil it will not be amiss.

GOOSBERRY JELLY.

PUT them into hot water, and keep on a flow fire till they rife on the furface of the water; then take them off the fire, and pour a little cold water in the pan to cool it; and to bring them to their proper green, put a little vinegar and falt to it; in about half an hour after drain them off this water into cold a moment; drain again off this fecond, and mix with as much weight of fugar, third degree; boil a little while till the fugar is again to the fame degree; take care to fkim it, and fift it through a fieve and put it in glaffes.

N. B. When you make any kind of fruit jelly, care fhould be taken not to let any of the feeds from the fruit fall into your jelly, nor fqueeze your fruit too near, for that will prevent your jelly from being fo tranfparent. It is alfo a great fault to boil any kind of jellies too high, as it makes them of a dark colour. Obferve to keep all wet fweetmeats in a dry cool place, for a wet damp place will make them mould, and a hot place will dry up their virtue, and make them candy; it muft alfo be remarked that many fweetmeats are fpoilt by the negligence in tying them down.

BLACK CURRANT JELLY.

GATHER your currants when they are ripe and dry, pick them off their ftalks, and put them in a large ftew pot, to every ten quarts of currants put a quart of water, tye a paper over them, and fet them in a cool oven for two hours, then fqueeze them through a very thin cloth, to every pound of juice add a pound and a half of loaf fugar broken in fmall pieces, ftir it gently till the fugar is melted; when it boils fkim it well, let it boil pretty quick for half an hour,

hour over a clear fire, then pour it into pots for use.

APPLE JELLY.

PEEL and slice golden pippins, according to what quantity of Jelly is required; boil with a little water, a lemon sliced; when boiled to a marmalade, sift the juice through a pretty fine sieve; the proportion is about a pint of this juice to a pound of sugar, of the eleventh degree; simmer it together on a slow fire, till it quits the spoon clean, by dropping it out of it; then it is fit to put into pots or glasses. Other sorts of apples also serve for jelly, done in a different manner; peel any kind of sharp apples, and cut in slices as the last; wash them in several waters; then boil in a good deal of water, the pot covered, untill the water is much reduced, and becomes gluish; strain it in a thin linen cloth; measure the decoction;

coction; and refine as much clarified sugar to the twelfth degree, and pour the juice in it gently; boil a moment, then take it off the fire and scim it, then boil it again till it comes to the same consistency as the last; prove it in the same manner.

How to make fruit Jams.

A FINE RASPBERRY JAM.

TAKE raspberries full ripe, bruise them fine, add a gill of the juice of currants and pass them through a sieve, to take out all the seeds; to every pound of pulp put a pound of double refined sugar pounded, boil it to a proper thickness, put into small pots or glasses, paper * it down according to the receipt for currant jelly; and keep it in a dry place. If you perceive it does not keep, boil it again, and add some more sugar to it.

* The proper papers for these uses are outside demy.

RED RASPBERRY JAM.

YOUR raspberries must be gathered when the sound ones are ripe and dry; pick them very carefully from the stalks, crush in a bowl with a silver or wooden spoon, pewter is apt to turn them a purple colour; as soon as you have done that, strew them in their own weight of loaf sugar, and half their weight of currant juice, baked and strained as for jelly, then set them over a clear slow fire, boil them half an hour, skim them well, and keep stirring them all the time, then put them into pots or glasses, with papers over them, and keep them for use.

N. B. As soon as you have got your berries, strew in your sugar, do not let them stand long before you boil them, and it will preserve their flavour

WHITE RASPBERRY JAM.

TAKE care to let your raspberries be dry and full ripe, (their flavour being at that time in its highest perfection) crush them fine, and to every pound of pulp add thereto the same weight of loaf sugar, and half their weight of the juice of white currants, boil them half an hour over a clear slow fire, skim them well, and put them into pots or glasses, tie them down with papers, and keep them dry for use.

N. B. Strew in your sugar as in the red raspberry Jam.

ANOTHER RASPBERRY JAM.

PRESS out the juice from the raspberries, and to every pound of raspberries take one pound of sugar; first dry the raspberries in a pan over the fire, but keep them stirring lest they burn;

put

put in your sugar, incorporate them well together, and fill your glasses or pots, covering them with thin white paper close to the jam, whilst it is hot, and when cold tie them over with other paper.

RED STRAWBERRY JAM.

GATHER the scarlet strawberries very ripe, bruise them very fine, and put to them a little juice of strawberries, beat and sift their weight in sugar, strew it among them, and put them in the preserving pan, set them over a clear flow fire, skim them, and boil them twenty minutes, then put them in pots or glasses for use.

GREEN GOOSBERRY JAM.

TAKE the green walnut goosberries when they are full grown, but not ripe, cut them in two and pick out the seeds, then put them in a pan of water, green them as you do the goosberries

ries, in imitation of hops, and lay them on a sieve to drain, then beat them in a marble mortar with their weight of sugar, then take a quart of goosberries, boil them to mash in a quart of water, then squeeze them, and to every pint of liquor put a pound of fine loaf sugar, boil and skim it, then put in your green goosberries, boil them till they are very thick, clear, and a pretty green, then put them in glasses for use.

CHERRY JAM.

TAKE twelve pounds of stoned cherries, boil them, break them as they boil; and when you have boiled all the juice away, and can see the bottom of the pan, put in three pounds of sugar finely beaten, stir it well, and let them have two or three boils; then put them in pots or glasses.

APRICOT JAM.

TAKE two pounds of apricots pared, and a pint of codling jelly, boil them very fast together till the jelly is almost wasted; then put to it a pound and a half of fine sugar, and boil it very fast till it jellies; put it into pots or glasses. You may make fresh clear cakes with this, and pippin jelly, in the Winter.

A method to make all sorts of Light, Seed, and other Cakes.

IT may not be improper to observe, that before you proceed to make any sort of cakes, that care should first be taken to have all your ingredients ready before you begin, then beat your eggs well, and not leave them till you have finished the cakes, for by such neglect, they would go back, and your cakes would not be light; if your cakes are to have butter in, take care you beat it to a fine cream before you put in your sugar,

gar, for if you beat it twice the time after it will not anfwer fo well.

A WHITE CURRANT CAKE.

TO two pounds of flour well dried, take a pound of fugar beat and fifted, one pound of butter, a quarter of an ounce of mace, the fame of nutmegs, fixteen eggs, two pounds and a half of currants, picked and wafhed, half a pound of candied lemon, the fame of fweet almonds, half a pint of fack or brandy, three fpoonfulls of orange flower water, beat your butter to a cream, put in your fugar, beat the whites of your eggs half an hour, mix them with your fugar and butter, then beat your yolks half an hour, mix them with your whites, it will take two hours beating put in your flower a little before your oven is ready, mix your currants and all your other ingredients lightly in, juft when you put it in your tin. Two hours will bake it.

A POUND CAKE.

SET a pound of flour before the fire to dry, and then let it stand to be cold; beat a pound of butter in a pan one way, till it is like a thick cream, beat up twelve eggs, (leaving out six whites) strain them into the butter, with a pound of sugar sifted, and a few carraways, stir these well together, then dust in the flour, and with a pudding stirrer, beat it very well for an hour; butter a pan, and bake it an hour in a quick oven.

For a change you may add currants instead of carraways.

COMMON SMALL CAKES.

TO a pound of flour, put a pound of butter, six eggs, (leaving out three whites) to three quarters of a pound of sugar powder, a glass of water, a

little

little lemon peel, chopped very fine, dried orange flowers; work it well together; then cut it in pieces, of what bigness you please, to bake, and glaze them with sugar.

TO MAKE A SEED CAKE THE NUNS WAY.

TO four pounds of the finest flour, add three pounds of double refined sugar beat and sifted; mix this with the flour, and set it before the fire to dry; beat up four pounds of nice fresh butter to a cream, break three dozen of eggs (leaving out sixteen whites) and beat them up very well, with a tea cup full of orange flower water, strain them into the butter, and beat them well therewith; take the flour and sugar, and mix in six ounces of carraway seeds; put these ingredients to the butter and eggs by degrees, beating all continually for two hours: Butter a hoop, and bake it three hours in a moderate oven. If you

you please, you may add two or three grains of ambergrease.

RATAFIA CAKES.

TAKE half a pound of sweet almonds, the same quantity of bitter, blanch, and beat them fine in orange, rose, or clear water, to keep them from oiling, pound and sift a pound of fine sugar, mix it with your almonds, have ready very well beat the whites of four eggs, mix them lightly with the almonds and sugar, put it in a preserving pan, and set it over a moderate fire, keep stirring it quick one way until it is pretty hot; when it is a little cool, roll it in small rolls and cut it in thin cakes, dip your hands in flour and shake them on it, give them each a light tap with your finger, put them on sugar papers, and sift a little fine sugar over them just as you are putting them into a slow oven.

SAVOY

SAVOY CAKES.

TAKE an equal weight of eggs and sugar; separate the yolks and whites; put the sugar to the yolks, with some lemon peel finely chopped, powder of orange flowers, or a spoonful of the water; beat up this very well together, and also the whites, which you mix with the yolks, stirring continually, and half as much weight of flour, as you used of eggs; pour it in the vessel you intend to bake it in, well rubbed with butter; bake it in a soaking oven, about an hour and a half; if it is of a good colour, you may serve it without garnishing; and if not, as it may be too brown, or two pale, glaze it with a white sugar glaze, as directed in almond paste croquante, or with any other colours, as directed in the last.

A COMMON SEED CAKE.

TAKE two pounds of flour, rub into it half a pound of powder sugar, one ounce of carraway
seeds

seeds beaten, have ready a pint of milk, with half a pound of butter melted in it, and two spoonfuls of new barm, make it up into a paste, set it on the fire to rise, flour your tin, and bake it in a quick oven.

TO MAKE CREAM CAKES.

BEAT the whites of nine eggs to a stiff froth, then stir it gently with a spoon, for fear the froth should fall, and grate in the rinds of two lemons, to every white of an egg, shake in softly a spoonful of double refined sugar sifted fine, lay a wet sheet of paper on a tin, and drop the froth in little lumps on it with a spoon, a small distance from each other, and sift a good quantity of sugar over them, set them in an oven after brown bread, make the oven close up, and the froth will rise, when they are just coloured they are baked enough, take them out and put two bottoms together, and lay them on a sieve, then set them

them in a cool oven to dry. You may lay raspberry jam, or any other sort of sweetmeat between them before you close the bottom together to dry.

TO MAKE A FINE SAFFRON CAKE.

A Receipt practised by Mrs. GLASS.

TAKE a quarter of a peck of fine flour, a pound and a half of fresh butter, a quarter of an ounce of mace and cinnamon together, beat fine, and mix the spice in the flour. Set on a quart of milk to boil, break the butter in, and stir it till the milk boils; take off all the butter, and a little of the milk; mix with the flour a pound of sugar beat fine, a penny-worth of saffron made into a tincture; take a pint of yeast that is not bitter, and stir it well into the remainder of the milk; beat up six eggs very well, and put to the yeast and milk, strain it to the flour, with some rose-water, and the tincture of saffron;

saffron; beat up all together with your hands lightly, and put it into a hoop or pan well buttered. It will take an hour and an half in a quick oven. You may make the tincture of saffron with the rose water.

TO MAKE A BRIDE CAKE MRS. RAFFALD's WAY

TAKE four pounds of fine flour well dried, four pounds of fresh butter, two pounds of loaf sugar, pound and sift fine a quarter of an ounce of mace, the same of nutmegs, to every pound of flour put eight eggs, wash four pounds of currants, pick them well and dry them before the fire, blanch a poundd of sweet almonds (and cut them length-way very thin) a pound of citron, one pound of candied orange, the same of candied lemon, half a pint of brandy; first work the butter with your hand to a cream, then beat in your sugar a quarter of an hour, beat the whites of your eggs to a very strong froth, mix them

them with your sugar and butter, beat your yolks half an hour at least, and mix them with your cake, then put in your flour, mace, and nutmeg, keep beating it well till your oven is ready, put in your brandy, and beat your currants and almonds lightly in, tie three sheets of paper round the bottom of your hoop to keep it from running out, rub it well with butter, put in your cake, and lay your sweet-meats in three lays, with cake betwixt every lay, after it is risen and coloured, cover it with paper before your oven is stopped up; it will take three hours baking.

TO MAKE ALMOND ICEING FOR THE BRIDE CAKE.

BEAT the whites of three eggs to a strong froth, beat a pound of Jordan almonds very fine with rose water, mix your almonds with the eggs lightly together, a pound of common loaf sugar beat fine, and put in by degrees, when your

cake

cake is enough, take it out and lay your icing on, and put it in to brown.

A FASHION CAKE.

MIX a handful of flour with a pint of good cream, half a pound of beef-suet, melted and sifted, a quarter of a pound of sugar-powder, half a pound of raisins stoned and chopped, dried flowers of orange, a glass of brandy, a little coriander and salt; bake it as all other cakes, about an hour, and glaze or garnish it.

RICE CAKE.

TAKE what quantity of rice you think proper; boil it in good broth, and some hog's-lard; when it is cold, mix it with as much flour as rice, a good deal of butter, some eggs, and salt; make a good puff-paste of it; and make hot cakes of what shape and bigness you please with it; rub them over with eggs, before baking, to give them a good colour.

TO MAKE RICE CAKE ANOTHER WAY.

TAKE fifteen eggs, leave out one half of the white, beat them exceeding well near an hour with a whisk, then beat the yolks half an hour, put to your yolks ten ounces of loaf sugar sifted fine, beat it well in, then put in half a pound of rice flour, a little orange water or brandy, the rinds of two lemons grated, then put in your whites, beat them all well together for a quarter of an hour, then put them in a hoop, and set them in a quick oven for half an hour.

BEAN CAKES.

TAKE weight for weight of fine sugar and blanched almonds cut in long narrow slices; slice some preserved orange, lemon, and citron peel; then beat the white of a new laid egg, with a little orange-flower water, to a high froth; put so much of the froth into the sugar as will just wet it, and with the point of a knife build up your almonds, piling it round as high as you can upon a wafer; let some ambergrease be in your sugar, and bake them after the manner of a manchet.

TO MAKE GUM CAKES.

TAKE gum tragacanth, commonly called gum dragon, let it lie all night in rose water till it is dissolved, have double-refined sugar beaten and seered, and mix your gum and sugar together; make it up into paste, then roll some up plain, and some with herbs and flowers; all the paste must be kept separately our herbs and flowers must be beat small before you make them into paste; but you may use the juice of the flowers and herbs only; I use sweet marjoram, red roses, clove-gilly-flowers, and blue-bottle berries, all clipped from the white again, for two colours will not do well; so roll; so roll them up, and cut them the bigness of a sixpence, but in what fashion you please, minding that they are rolled very thin.

TO MAKE HONEYCOMB CAKES.

TAKE your sugar and boil it to a candy-height then put in your flowers, which must be cut; have little papers with four corners ready; then drop some of your candy on the papers, take them off when ready, and if they are rightly done they will look full of holes like honeycombs.

HOW TO MAKE LEMON CAKES.

TAKE the best coloured lemons, scrape out the blacks, and grate off the peel clean; put the peel into a strainer; wet what sugar you think will serve and boil it to a candy-height; then take it off and put in your lemon peel;

when it boils take it off, squeeze in a litttle lemon juice, and drop them on buttered plates or papers; you may put in musk or ambergrease if you please.

TO MAKE LEMON, ORANGE, AND FLOWER CAKES.

TAKE sugar finely seered, and wet it with the juice of orange, or any flowers you fancy; there must be no more juice than will make your paste stiff and thick; set it upon the fire, when it begins to boil drop it in little cakes, and they will come off presently; scurvigrass done thus is good against the scurvy; if it boils you will spoil it.

VIOLET CAKES.

BEAT your sugar wherein gum hath been steeped, put in the violets and the juice, and so work it well together with seered sugar, and dry them in a stove.

HOW TO MAKE WORMWOOD CAKES.

TAKE one pound of double-refined sugar sifted, mix it with three or four eggs well beat, and drop in as much chemical oil of wormwood as you please; drop them on papers, and you may have them of various colours by pricking them with a pin and filling the small holes with such colours; you must keep your colours separate in small gallypots; for red, take a dram of cochineal, some cream of tartar, and as much allum; tie them up severally in little bits of fine cloth, and put them to steep in a glass of water two or three hours; when you want the colours press the bags in the water, and mix some of it in a little white of egg and sugar; use saffron for the yellow, prepared as the red; for green, mix blue with the saffron; for blue, put powder-blue in water.

HOW TO MAKE CAKES OF FLOWERS.

BOIL double-refined sugar to a candy-heigth, and then strew in your flowers and let them boil once up; then with your hand lightly strew in a little double-refined sugar sifted, and then be as quick as you can to put it into your little pans made of card, and pricked full of holes at the bottom; you must set the pans on a cushion, and when they are cold take them out

LIQUORICE CAKES.

TAKE hysop and red-rose water, of each half a pint, half a pound of green liquorice, the outside scraped off, and then beat with a pestle; put to it half a pound of annifeeds, and steep it all night in the water; boil it with a gentle fire till the taste is well out of the

the liquorice; strain it, put to it three pounds of liquorice powder, and set it on a gentle fire till it is come to the thickness of cream; take it off, and put to it half a pound of white sugar-candy seered very fine; beat this together as you do biscuit, for at least three hours, and never suffer it to stand still; as you beat it you must strew in double-refined sugar finely seered, at least three pounds; half an hour before it is finished, put in half a spoonful of gum-dragon steeped in orange-flower water; when it is very white then it is beat enough; roll it up with white sugar, and if you will have it perfumed must put in a pastil or two.

ALMOND CAKES.

TAKE a pound of double refined sugar finely seered, a quarter of a pound of the best almonds laid in cold water all night and blanched; take the white of an egg, put to it a spoonful of rose-water, and beat it to the whiteness of snow, letting it stand half an hour; beat your almonds, putting thereto a spoonful of rose-water, a little at once, and the same with the egg; when the almonds are well beat, put the sugar in by degrees, and minding you wet not the paste too much whilst you roll out the cakes; you must continue beating till all be used, and when your cakes are made, lay them severally on papers with some seered sugar over them; bake them in an oven as hot as for your sugar cakes.

TO MAKE ALMOND LOAVES.

BEAT a pound of almonds very fine, mix them well with three quarters of a pound of sifted sugar, set them over the fire, keep them stirring till they are stiff, and put in the rind of a lemon grated very fine; make them up in little loaves, shake them very well in the whites of

eggs

eggs beat to a very stiff froth, that the eggs may hang about them; then put them in a pan with a pound of fine sifted sugar; divide them if they stick together, and add more sugar, till they begin to be smooth and dry; and when you put them on papers to bake, shake them in a pan that is just wet with white of eggs, to make them have a gloss; bake them after biscuits, on papers and tin plates.

TO MAKE ALL SORTS OF SUGAR PASTE.

SIFT your sugar through a lawn sieve, then sift some starch as fine; to a pound of sugar put a quarter of a pound of starch; make it of what colour you please, into a stiff paste; putting thereto gum-dragon well steeped in orange-flower-water; beat it well in a mortar, and make it in knots or shells in a mould or moss, with rubbing it through an hair sieve: the red must be coloured with carmine; the yellow with gumboodge,

boodge, steeped in water, and put to the gum; the green is made yellow with gum, putting to it stone-blue steeped in water; the brown with chocolate, and the blue with smalt.

TO MAKE BEANED BREAD.

BLANCH half a pound of almonds, slice them thin the long way, lay them in rose-water all night; then drain them from the water, and set them by the fire, stirring them till they are a little dry and very hot; then put to them fine sugar sifted, enough to hang about them. (They must not be so wet as to make the sugar like paste; nor so dry, but that the sugar may hang together.) Then lay them in lumps on wafer-paper, and set them on papers in an oven, after puffs, or any very cool oven that pies have been baked in.

TO MAKE LITTLE ROUND RATAFIA PUFFS.

TAKE half a pound of kernels, or bitter-almonds, beat very stiff, and a pound and a half of sifted sugar; make it up to a stiff paste with white of eggs whipped to a froth; beat it well in a mortar, and make it up in little loaves; then bake them in a very cool oven, on paper and tin-plates.

TO MAKE BROWN WAFERS.

TAKE half a pint of milk and half a pint of cream, and put to it half a pound of brown sugar; melt and strain it through a sieve; take as much fine flour as will make one half of the milk and cream very stiff, then put in the other half; stir it all the while, that it may not be in lumps; then put in two eggs well beaten, a little sack, some mace shred fine, two or three cloves beaten: bake in irons.

PUFF CAKES.

MAKE some fine puff paste, roll it as thin as a crown piece, take a dish of the bigness of the cake you design to make, and place the same over your paste which you cut round. Being thus cut, put it on a sheet of paper, or upon a tin plate; then make another round piece of paste in the same manner, cutting it in what figures you please. Fill the first abbess either with a marmalade of apricots, or apples, or with a cream of pistachio's, and cover it with your abbess cut out into figures. Then bake your cake, and being done strew some fine sugar over it, and glaze it with a red hot fire shovel. Put it in its dish, and serve it up either hot or cold, if it is filled with cream, serve it up always hot.

A LISBON CAKE.

IN order to make this cake, get four or five pounds of fine flour, and make a good puff paste; that being done, roll it as thin as a half crown piece. Then put over it a dish of the bigness of the cake you design to make, cut your paste round it, and put this piece of paste so cut round upon a sheet of paper. Cut out in the same manner seven or eight abbesses more, cutting one of them into several figures, to be placed on the top of your cake. This being done, let them be baked separately, then glaze the abbess cut out into figures, and make your cake as follows: Put over one of these abbesses a laying of apricot marmalade; then over this another abbess with a laying of jelly of currants; again, another abbess over the last with jelly of gooseberries. Continue after the same manner to place the rest of your abbesses,

abbesses, putting between them your several layings of preserved raspberries, apple jelly, &c. placing on the top your figured and glazed abbess, so that the rest may not be seen: To which purpose, your cake must be glazed with a white glaze, a green glaze, and a cochineal colour glaze, that it may appear no more than one abbess. Make the glaze thus, *viz.* beat together in an earthen vessel with a wooden spoon about a pound of powder sugar, the white of two eggs, and the juice of half a lemon. If this mixture proves to be too thin, put some more sugar in it; then divide this composition into three parts: in the first, put nothing, but leave it white as it is; in the second, put a little cochineal, to make it red; and the third green, with some juice of spinage. Glaze your cake from top to bottom, first, with a streak of your white composition, then with a streak of the red, and afterwards with a streak of the green; following the same order till your cake is entirely glazed.

glazed. Then to dry your icing, put your cake for a little while, in a warm oven, or before the fire turning it round now and then. Your cake being as it should be, you lay it in its dish, and serve it up. It may be made as small or as large as you please.

SWORD KNOTS.

MAKE a second-best paste, and roll it very thin; cut it in thongs like ribbons, some with a knife, and some with a dented paste cutter, to make the scollop; fold them like a sword knot; wet the paste with eggs, where it should join together; bake them on a baking plate; and when ready to serve, garnish with currant jelly, apricot marmalade, frothed cream, or any thing else.

A CAKE CALLED PUIS D'AMOUR.

MAKE a puff paste, roll it into the thickness of a crown piece, and put it round a dish as before; put this first abbess upon a tin plate, then take another dish a thumb's breadth smaller than the first, and cut round it a second abbess; cut out of the middle of it, a piece of six inches in circumference, more or less, according to the bigness of your cake. This being done, put this last abbess over the first, and make with some of the same paste four SS, the bigness you think fit, at least four inches long. Let all be dried in the oven; then strow some sugar over your cake, glaze it with a red hot fire shovel. The four SS must be glazed all over. Make with paste a little chain of the length of four or five thumbs, like chain of a well, which must be baked, and glazed like the rest. Make likewise five small cakes

cakes of the bigness of a large apple with a paste, commonly called in French, *Petit choux gros*. These five small cakes are to be made in imitation of pales; and when baked, are to be filled up with currant jelly, or marmalade of apricots, spliting a corner without parting them. Then rub these small cakes with melted butter, strew them with sugar, and glaze them with a red hot fire shovel. The whole being ready, dish up your cake, and fill up the middle of it with some jelly of currants, or marmalade of apricots. Then warm some caramel in a stew-pan, in which you dip both ends of your SS, placing them upright or cross ways on your *Puis d'Amour*; so that one end of each may touch the top of the other. This done, dip likewise in your caramel the end of your chain, laying the same over the top of your SS, so that it may imitate the nature of a chain and pale of a well. After this, put one of your little cakes in the middle on the top of your well, and

and the other four between the intervals of your SS, and serve it up. You may make it as large or as little as you please.

SMALL CAKES OF PUIS d'AMOUR.

ROLL your puff paste of the same thickness as that before, cut it in abbesses of the bigness of the top of a wine glass, with a dented jagging iron, place them upon a tin plate: then make as many more abbesses about the sixth part smaller than the former; cut out of the middle of a round piece the breadth of a six-pence, more or less, according to the bigness of the *Puis d'Amour* you design to make; then put these abbesses over the first, keeping the small round pieces cut off to be baked with the rest; and when done, sweeten them with sugar: glaze it with a red hot fire shovel. Then pour in some jelly of currants or marmalade of apricots, then close them with

with the small round piece cut out. Dish up your cakes, and serve them up.

A CAKE ROLLED UP IN THE FORM OF A SNAIL.

GET some puff paste and cream made after the same manner, as in the article of cream tarts or franchipane; you may make it either white or green. Spread your paste the length of one or two yards, of the breadth of four or six fingers, and about the thickness of two crown pieces. Put your cream in the middle of the whole length of it, and close your paste so that your cream may not run out, and make it in the shape of a large sausage. This being done, put it on paper well buttered, turning it round to imitate the form of a snail, and rub it with beaten eggs. Bake it in a moderate oven and glaze it.

A CAKE CALLED FEUILLAN-TINE.

FOR this cake use the same sort of cream as in the foregoing article. Make an abbess over a sheet of paper, and put pour cream in it to make it finer; make round it an ornamental border of the same paste, making the same ornaments on the top. This being done, rub it with beaten eggs, and put it in the oven. When baked, you must glaze it with sugar through a red hot fire shovel; and serve it up either hot or cold.

A CRACKLING CAKE IN THE SHAPE OF A CROWN.

THIS is generally made with paste for a croquante, with which make some slips, which you

you put into a stew pan, imitating as much as possible the form of a crown, either imperial or any other. Colour it, and set it to bake. When baked, rub it with sweetmeats of divers colours, and strew over this small coloured sugar plumbs. Serve it up over a bottom like that of a croquante, with sweetmeats of divers colours garnished, provided it be broken through, and looks like a crown.

A CAKE CALLED CROQUANTE DE FEUILLETAGE.

MAKE an abbess of puff paste, put it in the bottom of a stew pan, or of a baking pan, and cut it into what shape you please. Let it be half baked, then sugar it, and particularly the slits of the puff. Put it into the oven again, do not let it be out of your sight; let it glaze well, take it out, let it be half cold, take it off without breaking, make another abbess with some of the same puff-paste, of the same bigness as the other, and let it be baked: then dish it up, rub it with jelly of currants or other sweetmeats, put over it your glazed abbess, and serve it up.

TO MAKE ORANGE CLEAR CAKES

TAKE the best pippins, pare them into as much water as will cover them, and boil them to a mash; then press out the jelly upon a sieve, and strain it through a bag, adding juice of oranges to give it an agreeable taste; to every pound of jelly take one pound and a quarter of loaf sugar, boil it till it cracks, and then put in the jelly and the rind of a grated orange or two; stir it up gently over a slow fire, till all is incorporated together; then take it off, and fill your clear cake glasses; what scum arises on the top, you must carefully take off before they are cold; then put them into a stove, and when you find them begin to cruſt upon the upper ſide, turn them out upon ſquares of glaſſes and put them to dry again; when they begin to have a tender candy, cut them into quarters or what pieces you pleaſe, and let them dry till hard; then turn them on ſieves, and, when thoroughly dry, pour them into your boxes.

TO MAKE ORANGE FLOWER PASTE.

BOIL one pound of the leaves of orange flowers very tender; then take two pounds of double refined ſugar in fine powder, and when you have bruiſed the flowers to a pulp, ſtir in the ſugar by degrees, over a ſlow fire, till all is in and well melted; then make little drops and dry them.

Puff Paste for all Sorts of Tarts made with Sweetmeats and Cream.

TO make this sort of paste good, take twelve pounds of fine flour, breaking six eggs in the hollow made in the middle, with about a pound of butter and an ounce of salt, if it is fresh butter, but if salt, then less salt will suffice. then wet your flour with cold water, make your paste no harder than your butter. Thus keep it a little while in a cool place; then take twelve pounds of butter, which you will work to take the water out, and having rolled your paste, spread your butter over it. Now turn over your paste, with the butter in it, roll it twice or thrice. then lay it by for a little while. If you design to make patty-pattees, roll your paste four or five times, and lay it in the bottom of your patty-pans.

The same is to be done with all sorts of pastry, except tarts, where the paste must be rolled once more, if you take twelve pounds of fine flower. The same proportion is to be observed with one pound as with twelve.

ANOTHER WAY TO MAKE PUFF PASTE.

PASTE made for raised crust is done with less butter, and firmer, and is done with warm water; let it rest some time, then raise it upon paper for puff paste; use about a pound of butter to a quarter of a pound of fine flour, and some salt, and cold water to work it.

A RICH PUFF PASTE.

MIX some fine flour with cold water, salt, one or two eggs; the paste ought to to be as soft as the butter it is made with; in winter soften the butter, with squeezing it in your hands; in summer,

mer, ice it; put butter according to judgment, to make it very rich, and work it with a rolling-pin several times, folding it in three or four folds each time: use it to any kind of pies, or small cakes.

ROYAL PASTE.

BOIL half a pint of water a moment, with a little sugar, a quarter of a pound of butter, a little fine rasped or grated lemon peel, a little salt; put flour to it, by little and little, to mix it well, and pretty thick; turn and stir it continually on the fire, until it quits the pan; take it off, and while it is warm, put eggs to it, one by one; mix it well, and put eggs, until it is come to the consistency of a paste, and sticks to the fingers.

QUEEN PASTE.

IT is done after the same manner as the last, except you are to use cream, instead of water;

it will have a richer taste, but will not be so light.

PASTE SPANISH FASHION.

MAKE a hole in the middle of the flour; put salt to it, and half butter, and half fresh hog's lard; mix it with warm water; make it pretty firm, and let it rest; cut it in several pieces, and roll each as thin as possible, and rub each leaf with melted hog's lard; put all the pieces one upon another; roll them together; let it cool; cut it with a knife, to put to what use you please.

A PARTICULAR PASTE, TO BAKE OR FRY ANY THING IN IT.

MELT a little butter in a glass of water, and some fine rasped or grated lemon peel, and an egg; mix half as much powder sugar as flour,

flour; mix it, and work it with the above liquid; put flour enough to keep it firm.

RICE PASTE.

WORK some flour with a couple of eggs, and a little water; let it rest; have some rice boiled very tender, in good rich broth; when it is cold, pound it in a mortar with the ready prepared paste, and a little butter, until it is properly mixed: it will serve for any sorts of cakes, as all other paste.

A PUFF PASTE FOR TARTS OR PYES WITH FRUIT, PRESERVES, AND OTHER SWEET MEATS.

TAKE two handfuls of fine flour, put it on a clean table, make a hollow in the middle of your flour, put in an egg, with a bit of butter the bigness of an egg, and a little salt, if the butter is fresh. Wet the flour with cold water, let your

your paste be as stiff as your butter, then roll it, spread it over with butter, double the paste, roll it once or twice or more, till the butter is well mixed in the paste. Rowl it for an under-crust, put it in a baking-pan, then put in a marmalade either of preserved apples, cherries, apricots, goosberries, jelly, or any other sort; now roll your paste very thin, flour it, double it four or five times, then cut it into long and thin slices, place them on the top of your tarts in what shape you think fit; put round it a slip of the same paste, of about the breadth of a thumb, which slip pare off neatly. Your tart being done either in the oven or in a baking-pan with fire under and over, strew some sugar over it, glaze it with a red-hot fire-shovel, then dish it up, and serve it either hot or cold.

A TART

A TART WITH A MARMALADE OF APPLES.

PARE some apples, cut them in four, take out the cores, cut them in small bits, put them in a stew-pan over the fire with a little water, some sugar, and a stick of cinnamon. When turned to a marmalade, rasp or grate into it some green lemon peel, let it be of a fine flavour and cold. Roll out some puff paste, and put it into a baking-pan, as large as the tart you design to make; then put in your marmalade which you cover with paste, either cut into several forms, or in thin slips, doing the rest as in the article before.

Pippins are the best apples to make this sort of marmalade.

A BON

A BON CHRETIEN PEAR PYE
(CALLED A LA BONNE FEMME.)

SLIT in two some bon chrétien pears, take out the core, pare them. Put into an earthen pot some of the parings, put the apple over them, add a stick of cinnamon and some sugar, and a glass of red wine, with a little water; and cover the same with the rest of the parings. Cover your pot with some paste round, and let your pears be doing slowly during five or six hours, with fire under and over; then put some paste in the bottom of a baking-pan, as large as the dainty dish you design to serve up, making round it a crust the breadth of a thumb; and let the paste be not too thick. Put the pan in the oven, and when baked, glaze the paste. Your pears being done, place them in the pan, with their liquor, which must be of a lively red, strain it through a sieve, and pour it over them. If your
liquor

liquor is too thin, set it over again to thicken, then pour it over your pears. Serve it up either hot or cold.

TO MAKE TARTS.

TAKE apples, or pears, cut them in small quarters, and set them over the fire, with a piece of lemon peel, and some cinnamon; let them simmer in as much water as will cover them, till tender; and if you bake them in tin patty pans, butter them first, and lay over a thin paste; lay in some sugar, then the fruit, with three or four tea spoonfuls of the liquor they were simmered in; put in a little more sugar, and lid them over. If your tarts are made of apricots, green almonds, nectarines, or green plumbs, they must be scalded before you use them, and observe to put nothing to them but sugar, and as little water as possible; make use of the syrrup they were scalded in, in, as you did for your apples, &c. cherries currants, raspberries, and all ripe fruit need not be scalded; and if you make your tarts in china, or glass patties, lay the sugar at bottom, then the fruit with a little more sugar on the top; put no paste at the bottom, only lid them over, and bake them in a slack oven. You have receipts how to make crusts for tarts; mince pies must be baked in tin patties, that you may slip them out into a dish, and a puff paste is the best for them.

When you make sweetmeat tarts, or a crocant tart, lay in the sweetmeats, or preserved fruits either in glass or china patties that are small, for that purpose; lay a very thin crust on the top, and let them be baked no more than till your crust is nicely coloured, and that in a slow oven. If you would have a crocant tart for the middle of the table, or a side dish, have a glass, or china dish, of what size you please, and lay in the preserved

served fruits of different sorts, (you must have a round cover just the size of the inside of your dish) roll out a sugar crust, the thickness of an half crown, and lay over the cover; mark it with marking irons made on purpose for that use, of what shapes you please; then put the crust, with the cover, into a very slack oven, not to discolour it, only to have it crisp. When you take it out of the oven, loosen it from the cover very gently, and when quite cold, take it carefully off, and lay over your sweetmeats, and it being hollow, you will see the fruit through it. If the tart is not eaten, only take off the lid, and your sweetmeats may be put into the pots again.

A PEACH TART.

TAKE ripe peaches, slit them in two, pare them, take out the core, put in the bottom of a stew-pan some powdered sugar, place your peaches

peaches in it, put them over the fire, stir them now and then, make an under-crust with a border round it, the thickness of a thumb, and let it be baked; when done, put them in its dish, and your peaches being ready and pretty well coloured, turn them upside down in a dish, put them over your under crust. Put a little water in the stew-pan, where your peaches were on the fire, to make a little syrrup with the sugar remaining in it, and pour this liquor over your peaches, placing over them their kernels. This tart is served up either hot or cold.

ANOTHER PEACH-TART.

YOUR peaches being ready done in sugar, as those before, place them over the paste prepared for an under-crust, and let them either be baked in the oven, or under a cover with fire under and over. When done you will glaze

them

them with sugar, by means of a red-hot fire-shovel, and serve it up hot or cold.

A CREAM TART.

PUT in a Stew-pan two spoonfuls of fine flour, with the yolks of six eggs reserving the white of them. Mix your flower in a quart of milk, and season it with sugar and a stick of cinnamon, keep it stirring with a ladle, and put in a good lump of butter. Your cream being half done, put in some green lemon grated, some preserved lemon peel shred small with some bitter almond-biskets, let the whole be thoroughly done. When ready, let it be cold, then put an abbess of puff-paste in a baking pan with a border of paste, and put your cream over it, mix it with some orange flower-water and the white of eggs beaten up to snow; take care not to over-fill your custard, and let it be done either in the oven or under the cover of a

baking

baking pan, with fire under and over. When ready and glazed with fugar, by means of a red-hot fire-fhovel, ferve it up hot

Cream tarts are made after the fame manner.

ALMOND PYE.

GET a pound of fweet almonds fkinned, pound them well, moiften them now and then with the white of eggs. Beat up the white of eight eggs to fnow, mix four of their yolks with Savoy bifcuits, rafped green lemon-peel, preferved lemon peel cut fmall, and fome crifped orange flower, or orange flower-water. This done, take your almonds out of the mortar, mix them with the aforefaid ingredients, fugar it and fweeten it moderately, add the beaten white of eggs, put it over your abbefs with a border round ready done with puff-pafte in a baking pan, and let it be baked. The reft being done,

done, as said about those before, serve it up hot.

PISTACHIO TART.

GET a pound of pistachios scalded, pound them and do them as directed to be done with the almond-pye. Take three or four Savoy biscuits, moisten them a little with cream or milk, let them be handled like paste. Then mix them with the same things prescribed in the article of almond pye; doing the rest as is explained in the said article.

ANOTHER PISTACHIO TART.

YOUR pistachioes being scalded and pounded, mix them with some pastry cream; strew over them sugar, rasped green lemon-peel, and preserved lemon peel cut small; add the white of six eggs beaten up to snow; do the rest as before.

The above two compositions with pistachioes, are to be made use of with tarts, and in the following pastry.

A CHOCOLATE TART.

PUT two spoonfuls of fine flour in a stew-pan, with the yolks of six eggs, reserve their white, mix these with some milk, add a quarter of a pound of rasped chocolate with a stick of cinnamon, some sugar, a little salt, and some rasped green lemon-peel; and let them be a little while over the fire. After which put in a little preserved lemon peel cut small, and having tasted whether it has a fine flavour, let it cool. When cold, mix this with the reserved white of eggs beat up to snow doing the rest as directed in the other articles.

This composition, as also the marmalade made either with apples or with apricots, may be used with *tarts, feuillantines, genoises, cakes,* &c.

ANOTHER CHOCOLATE TART.

PUT a spoonful of rice flower, and a little salt into a pan, together with the yolks of five eggs, a little milk, and mix them well together; then add a pint of cream, and sugar according to your discretion; set it all to boil over a stove, taking care that it do not curdle: mean while grate some chocolate into a plate, dry it a little before the fire, and when your cream is boiled, take it off the fire, mix your chocolate well with it, and set it by to cool; sheet a tart-pan, put in your cream and bake it; when it is baked, glaze it with powdered sugar and a red-hot shovel so serve it.

AN ALMOND TART.

RAISE an excellent good paste, six corners, and an inch deep, and take some blanched almonds, very finely beaten with rose-water;

take a pound of sugar to a pound of almonds, some grated bread, nutmeg, a little cream with strained spinnage, as much as will colour the almonds green. So bake it with a gentle hot oven, not shutting the door. Draw it, and stick it with orange citron.

A COWSLIP TART.

TAKE the blossoms of a gallon of cowslips, mince them exceedingly small, and beat them in a mortar; put to them a handful or two of grated *Naples* biscuit, and about a pint and a half of cream, boil them a little over the fire, then take them off, and beat them in eight eggs with a little cream; if it does not thicken, put it over again till it does; take heed that it do not curdle. Season it with sugar, rose-water, and a little salt; bake it in a dish or little open tartest. It is best to let your cream be cold before you stir in the eggs.

ORANGE OR LEMON TART.

TAKE fix large lemons, and rub them very well with falt, and put them in water for for two days, with a handful of falt in it; then change them into frefh water every day, (without falt) for a fortnight, then boil them two or three hours till they are tender, then cut them into half quarters, and then cut them three corner ways, as thin as you can: take fix pippins pared, cored, and quartered, and a pint of fair water. Let them boil till the pippins break; put the liquor to your orange or lemon, and half the pippins well broken, and a pound of fugar. Boil thefe together a quarter of an hour, then put it in a gallipot, and fqueeze an orange in it: if it be a lemon tart, fqueeze a lemon, two fpoonfuls is enough for a tart. Your patty-pans muft be fmall and fhallow. Put fine puff-pafte, and very thin; a little while will bake it.

Just as your tarts are going into the oven, with a feather, or brush, do them over with melted butter, and then sift double refined sugar over them; and this is a pretty icing on them.

APRICOT TARTS.

THESE tarts may be made with apricots of any ripeness, but if your fruit is not ripe enough, boil them a little while in water; (observing first to cut them in two, and break the stones, if possible, so as not to bruise the kernels) then drain them very well, and put them in the paste with sugar according to judgment, a few bits of preserved lemon, and half a kernel upon each piece; cover it with the same sort of paste, and throw a little powder-sugar over it to give it a glaze, which it will take in baking.

PLUMB

PLUMB TARTS.

THE same management, with regard to boiling, must be observed with green or hard plumbs, and if large, must be split also; put a good quantity of sugar, both under and over: use the same paste as the last, with the topcrust the same, and glaze it to give it a better look on the table; in regard to glazing any sorts of tarts, it is no farther necessary than agreeable, as many people like the crust, without its being glazed

N. B. The kernels are seldom made use of.

A FASHION TART.

SCALD spinnage in boiling water, and drain it very well to chop; then stew it in butter and cream, with a little salt, and sugar, few small bits of dried comfit-citron, and few drops of orange flower water; use either the finest puff paste, or the second.

ANGELICA

ANGELICA TARTS.

TAKE the stalks, peel them, cut them into little pieces, pare some golden pippins or nonpareils, of each an equal quantity; first take away the parings of the apples and the coars, boil them in as much water as will cover them, with a little lemon peel and fine sugar till it is like a very thin syrrup, then strain it off, and set the syrrup on the fire again with the angelica, let boil about ten minutes, then when the crust is ready, lay a sliced apple and a layer of angelica, so on till the pattypans are full, and bake them, filling them first with the syrrup.

GREEN GOOSBERRY TARTS.

YOU may either use them whole, or make a marmalade of them, with a good syrrup; this last is recommended as the best method; for by this

this means you can judge easily how sweet they are, and ought to be, to please; for the marmalade, they ought to be stoned, when they are pretty large.

TO MAKE MINCED MEAT.

PARE and core pippins, till you have got a pound; add of beef suet a pound, and raisins stoned half a pound; chop these very fine; take candied orange, lemon, and citron, one ounce of each, a pound of currants washed clean, and rubbed in a cloth till dry; half a pound of sugar, and a little salt; cinnamon and mace a quarter of an ounce of each, finely beaten, and a quarter of a pint of red wine; shred the sweetmeats, but not very small; then mix all very well together, and put it close down into a pot for use.

When you make your pies, squeeze a little orange into them.

TO MAKE MINCED PIES ANOTHER WAY.

PARE and core two pounds of golden pippens; two pounds of suet clean picked, and two pounds of raisins of the sun stoned; chop these separately very fine add two pounds of currants washed, dried, and rubbed very clean in a cloth, put these ingredients together, into a large pan, shew in half an ounce of cinnamon beaten fine, a pound of lump sugar pounded, the peel of a lemon cut fine, the juice of a Seville orange, a gill of sack, and a gill of brandy: Mix all these very well together; then put it down close in a pot, and lay over it writing paper dipped in brandy. When you make your pies, add sweetmeats to them, if you please; but you will find them exceedingly good without.

TO MAKE MINCED PIES FOR LENT.

BOIL six eggs hard, a dozen of golden pippens pared and cored, a pound of raisons of the sun stoned; chop these separately very fine; a pound of currants washed, cleaned, and rubbed in a cloth, two ounces of sugar pounded, an ounce of citron, and an ounce of candied orange, both cut small, a quarter of an ounce of beaten cinnamon, two cloves beat fine, and half a nutmeg grated, a gill of canary, and half a gill of brandy; squeeze in the juice of Seville orange; mix these all well together, and press them close down into a pot for use.

TO MAKE COMMON FRITTERS.

TAKE half a pint of ale and two eggs, beat in as much flower as will make it rather thicker than a common pudding, with nutmeg, and

and sugar to your taste, let it stand three or four minutes to rise; then drop them with a spoon into a pan of boiling lard, fry them a light brown, drain them on a sieve, serve them up with sugar grated over them, and wine sauce in a boat.

APPLE FRITTERS.

PARE the largest baking apples you can get, take out the core with an apple scraper, cut them in round slices, and dip them in batter, made as for common fritters, fry them crisp, serve them up with sugar grated over them, and wine sauce in a boat.

They are proper for a side dish for supper.

CLARY FRITTERS.

BEAT two eggs exceedingly well with one spoonful of cream, one of ratifia water,

one

one of loaf sugar, and two spoonfuls of flour, grate in half a nutmeg, have ready washed and dried clary leaves; dip them in the batter and fry them a nice brown; serve them up with quarters of Seville oranges laid round them, and good melted butter in a boat.

RASPBERRY FRITTERS.

GRATE two Naples biscuits, pour over them half a gill of boiling cream, when it is almost cold, beat the yolks of four eggs to a strong froth, beat the biscuits a little, then beat both together exceeding well, put to it two ounces of sugar, and as much juice of raspberry as will make it a pretty pink colour, and give it a proper sharpness, drop them into a pan of boiling lard, the size of a walnut; when you dish them up, stick bits of citron in some, and blanched almonds cut length-ways in others; lay round them green and yellow sweetmeats and
serve

serve them up. They are a pretty corner dish for either dinner or supper.

PLUMB FRITTERS WITH RICE.

GRATE the crumbs of a penny loaf, pour over them a pint of boiling cream, or good milk, let them stand four or five hours, then beat it exceedingly fine, put to it the yolks of five eggs, four ounces of sugar, and a nutmeg grated, beat them well together, and fry them in hog's lard, drain them on a sieve, and serve them up with white wine sauce under them.

N. B. You may put currants in if you please.

STRAWBERRY FRITTERS.

MAKE a paste with flour, a spoonful of fine oil, chopped lemon-peel, half whites of eggs beat up, and half white wine sufficient to one of loaf sugar, and two spoonfuls of flour, grate in half a nutmeg, have ready washed and dried clary leaves; dip them in the batter and fry them a nice brown; serve them up with quarters of Seville oranges laid round them, and good melted butter in a boat.

RASPBERRY FRITTERS.

GRATE two Naples biscuits, pour over them half a gill of boiling cream, when it is almost cold, beat the yolks of four eggs to a strong froth, beat the biscuits a little, then beat both together exceeding well, put to it two ounces of sugar, and as much juice of raspberry as will make it a pretty pink colour, and give it a proper sharpness, drop them into a pan of boiling lard, the size of a walnut; when you dish them up, stick bits of citron in some, and blanched almonds cut length-ways in others; lay round them green and yellow sweetmeats and serve

serve them up. They are a pretty corner dish for either dinner or supper.

PLUMB FRITTERS WITH RICE.

GRATE the crumbs of a penny loaf, pour over them a pint of boiling cream, or good milk, let them stand four or five hours, then beat it exceedingly fine, put to it the yolks of five eggs, four ounces of sugar, and a nutmeg grated, beat them well together, and fry them in hog's lard, drain them on a sieve, and serve them up with white wine sauce under them.

N. B. You may put currants in if you please.

STRAWBERRY FRITTERS.

MAKE a paste with flour, a spoonful of fine oil, chopped lemon-peel, half whites of eggs beat up, and half white wine sufficient to make it pretty soft, just fit to drop with a spoon; mix some large strawberries with it; and drop the bigness of a nutmeg in the hot fritter, as many as you propose to make; be careful to take them out, in the same manner as they are draining and glaze them with sugar.

RICE FRITTERS.

HAVING some rice, wash it in five or six several waters, and dry it very well before the fire: then beat it in a mortar very fine, and sift it through a lawn-sieve, that it may be very fine. You must have at least an ounce of it, then put it into a sauce-pan, just wet it with milk, and when it is well incorporated with it, add to it another pint of milk; set the whole over a stove or a very slow fire, and take care to keep it always moving; put in a little sugar, and some candied lemon-peel grated, keep it over the fire till it is almost come to the thickness of of a fine paste, flour a peel, pour it on it, and spread it abroad with a rolling pin. When it is quite cold cut it into little morsels, taking care that they stick not one to the other; flour your hands and roll up your fritters handsomely, and fry them. When you serve them up pour a little orange flower water over them and sugar. These make a pretty side dish; or are very pretty to garnish a side dish with.

ORANGE FRITTERS.

TAKE one or two preserved oranges, which you cut in as many pieces as you think proper; make a good thick batter, with sweet wine, and finish these as all others the same may be done with lemon, bergamotte, or any other fruits.

CURD FRITTERS.

HAVING a handful of curds, and a handful of flour, and ten eggs well beaten and strained, some sugar, cloves, mace and nutmeg beat, a little saffron; stir all well together, and fry them quick, and of a fine light brown.

OLIVE FRITTERS.

MAKE a thin puff-paste cut in small bits, and in each put a little boiled cream and mix a few pistachio nuts bruised in it; wet the borders with water or yolks of eggs, to pinch them close; fry them of a good colour; you may also glaze them brown or white; these are also done with apples, marmalade, or any other, either baked or fried.

FRITTERS ITALIAN FASHION.

BOIL a quarter of a pound of rice, very tender in milk; when it is pretty thick, put a little salt, some fine sugar, orange-flower preserved, and green chopped lemon-peel, a handful of flour, three whole eggs; mix it all very well; and add some currants, or couple of good apples, peeled and cut in small bits; butter a sheet of paper; and put this preparation upon it singly, with a spoon, each about the bigness of a large nutmeg; put this sheet of paper into your pan observing to have butter enough not to let them burn when they quit the paper, take it out and continue frying till they are of a good colour; take them out to drain upon a sieve; strew a little sugar powder upon; and serve them as hot as possible.

ENGLISH FASHION.

BEAT up six whole eggs, with a good handful of flour, salt, fine sugar, green lemon-peel, chopped, orange-flower water, macaroni-drops bruised, half a pint of good rich cream; rub the inside of a stew-pan with butter; and boil this preparation slowly, between two fires, without stirring it; when it is simmered thick enough, turn it over upon a dish, and let it cool to harden it; when you mean to use it, cut in small pieces, and fry it of a good colour: finish as the last.

ALMOND FRITTER.

POUND half a pound of sweet almonds, and six or eight bitter ones, orange-flowers, chopped lemon-peel, sugar in proportion, a handful of flour, two or three whites of eggs; pound all together some time, wih a few drops of water, or more whites of eggs, to make it of a a proper suppleness, to roll it in little balls; roll them in flour, to fry as force-meat bullets; strew a little fine sugar powder upon them when ready to serve

COURT CHEESECAKES.

BOIL a bit of butter in a little water and a little salt; thicken it with as much flour as it will take, stirring it on the fire constantly until it become quite a paste; then mix the eggs with it one by one, to make it almost as liquid as a thick batter; and mix some good cream cheese with it; bake it in good puff paste, coloured with yolks of eggs: serve hot or cold.

TO MAKE BAKED CUSTARDS.

BOIL a pint of cream with cinnamon, mace, and a bit of lemon peel; when cold, beat up four eggs, leaving out two whites, a little orange and rose water, a glass of sack, and a little nutmeg grated; sweeten it to your taste, mix them well together, and bake them in china cups, in an oven not too hot.

TO MAKE ALMOND CUSTARDS.

TAKE a pint of cream, beat a quarter of a pound of blanched almonds fine, with two spoonfuls of orange flower water, sweeten it to your taste; beat up the yolks of two eggs, and stir all together one way; boil it over a gentle clear fire till it is thick, then pour it into a cup and bake it.

TO MAKE A TANSEY.

BEAT ten eggs very well with a little salt, half a pound of loaf sugar, pounded, half a pint of spinnage juice, and a spoonful of the juice of tansey; mix them well together, and strain it to a quart of cream; grate in half a pound of Naples biscuits, and a nutmeg; add a quarter of a pound
of

of Jordan almonds blanched and beat fine, with a little rose water, and mix all well together; put it into a stew pan, with a piece of butter the bigness of a golden pippin. Set it over a slow charcoal fire; keep it stirring till it is hardened; then butter a dish very well, that will just hold it: Put in the tansey, bake it in a moderate oven taking care that it is not scorched. When it comes home, turn it upon a pye plate, cut Seville oranges in small quarters, and lay round it, and on the tansey, citron and orange peel cut thin, with double refined sugar laid in little heaps between.

If you have not Naples biscuits, grate seven ounces of the finest stale bread you have.

OF

and rose water, a glass of sack, and a little nutmeg grated; sweeten it to your taste, mix them well together, and bake them in china cups, in an oven not too hot.

TO MAKE ALMOND CUSTARDS.

TAKE a pint of cream, beat a quarter of a pound of blanched almonds fine, with two spoonfuls of orange flower water, sweeten it to your taste, beat up the yolks of two eggs, and stir all together one way; boil it over a gentle clear fire till it is thick, then pour it into a cup and bake it.

TO MAKE A TANSEY.

BEAT ten eggs very well with a little salt, half a pound of loaf sugar pounded, half a pint of spinnage juice, and a spoonful of the juice of tansey; mix them well together, and strain it to a quart of cream; grate in half a pound of Naples biscuits, and a nutmeg; add a quarter of a pound

of

of Jordan almonds blanched and beat fine, with a little rose water, and mix all well together; put it into a stew pan, with a piece of butter the bigness of a golden pippin. Set it over a slow charcoal fire; keep it stirring till it is hardened; then butter a dish very well, that will just hold it: Put in the tansey, bake it in a moderate oven taking care that it is not scorched. When it comes home, turn it upon a pye plate, cut Seville oranges in small quarters, and lay round it, and on the tansey, citron and orange peel cut thin, with double refined sugar laid in little heaps between.

If you have not Naples biscuits, grate seven ounces of the finest stale bread you have.

OF STRAWBERRIES AND ICED CREAMS.

MAKE an almond paste, as before directed put it in a baking dish, and raise a border as to any other sorts of paste; it requires but a short time to bake, and very little heat; just before you are ready to serve, put ice cream in it not very hard, and the strawberries upon it; this ice cream is made with a pint of good cream, and sugar sufficient to make it pretty sweet, a little orange flower water, two yolks of eggs; put it on the fire till it is ready to boil, stir it, to mix the eggs very well; when it is cold, put it in a mould to ice, as is explained in ice cream articles; you may also boil pistachio nuts in this cream, and sift it before icing.

CREAM CURD FOR CHEESECAKES.

TAKE a pint of cream, boil it with a little mace, cinnamon, and rose water, to make it sweet; when it is as cold as new milk, put in about half a spoonful of good runnet, and when it curds, serve it up in a cream dish.

QUEEN's CREAM.

BOIL a pint of cream to half reduced, with fine sugar, orange flower water; when half cold, mix it with six whites of eggs well beat up; bake it between two very moderate fires, and let it remain in its natural colour.

TO MAKE RHENISH WINE CREAM.

PUT over the fire a pint rhenish wine, a stick of cinnamon, and half a pound of sugar. While this is boiling, take seven yolks and whites of eggs, beat them well together with a whisk, till your wine is half driven in them, and your eggs to a fyrup; ftrike it very faft with the whifk till it comes to that thicknefs that you may lift it on the point of a knife, but be fure you let it not curdle; add to it the juice of a lemon, and orange flower water; fo pour it in your difh, and garnifh it with citron, fugar, or bifcuit, and ferve it up.

BURGUNDY CREAM.

WITH a pint of new milk boil a bit of lemon peel, orange flower water, a bit of fugar; and boil a quarter of a pound of rice in a little water, till it is tender and become thick; then add the milk to it, by a little and little, until all is boiled quite thick; fift it, and mix it well with fix or eight whites of eggs, well beat up; put it in the table difh: and bake it in a mild oven, or with a brazing pan cover; when ready to ferve, glaze it with a little ftrewed over it, and the falamander, or a hot fhovel, to catch flightly upon the fugar.

TO MAKE HARTSHORN CREAM.

TO four ounces of hartshorn shavings, boil three pints of water till they are reduced to half a pint, run it through a jelly bag, put to it a pint of cream, let it boil just up, then put it into jelly glasses, let it stand till it is cold, by dipping your glasses into scalding water it will slip out whole, then stick them all over with slices of almonds cut length ways: It eats well with white wine and sugar, like flummery.

TO MAKE SNOW CREAM.

TAKE a large deep dish, strew the bottom with fine sugar beat to powder; then fill it with strawberries; take some sprigs of rosemary, stick a large one in the middle, and several round about, to resemble a tree; then take a quart of the thickest cream you can get, and the whites of eight or ten eggs; then whisk it up for half

an

an hour, till you have made the froth very strong; let it stand ten minutes, and with a proper thing take off the froth, throw it over your tree, and cover your dish well with it; if you do it well, it makes a grand pile in a defert.

TO MAKE SPANISH CREAM.

TAKE three spoonfuls of flour of rice beat very fine; the yolks of three eggs, three spoonfuls of fair water, two spoonfuls of orange flower water, and mix them well together, then put to it one pint of cream, set it on a good fire, keeping it stirring till it is of a proper thickness, and then pour it into your cups.

TO MAKE POMPADOUR CREAM.

BEAT the whites of five eggs to a strong froth, put them into a tossing pan, with two spoonfuls of orange flower water, two ounces of sugar, stir it gently for three or four minutes,
then

then pour it into your dish, and pour good melted butter over it, and send it in hot.

It is a pretty corner dish for a second course at dinner.

ALMOND CREAM.

BLANCH almonds, bruise them small in a mortar, and strain them through a strainer with fair water; strain them again with thick milk, and with a quarter of a pound of sugar; put them into a pot, add a little salt, and set it over the fire; stir it well that it burn not to the pot; when it is boiled take it from the fire, cast a ladle of fair water into it, cover it with a dish, and let it stand; afterwards take a clean cloth of an ell long, let it be held strait and cast the cream upon it with a ladle, draw from under the cloth the water from the cream, pin the four corners together, and hang it up again.

CHOCOLATE CREAM.

TAKE half a pound of the best chocolate, cut or scraped, put to it as much water as will dissolve it, put in a very small, marble mortar, beat it very smooth, put in as much fine sugar as will sweeten it and add near a quart of cream; mill it, and as the froth rises lay it on a sieve, put the remaining part of your cream in posset glasses, and lay the frothed cream upon them.

PISTACHIO CREAM.

PEEL half a pound of pistachio nut-kernels, beat them very fine with a spoonful of brandy, put them into a tossing pan, with a pint of good cream and the yolks of two eggs beat fine, stir it gently over a very slow fire till it grows thick, put it into your plates; when it is cold, serve it up.

ANOTHER

ANOTHER WAY.

PEEL your piſtachios, beat them very fine in a marble mortar, boil them in cream; if it is not green enough add a little juice of ſpinnage, thicken it with eggs, ſweeten it to your palate, pour it into baſons and ſet it by till it is quite cold.

RASPBERRY CREAM.

TAKE the whites of ſeven eggs, and ſeven ſpoonfuls of raſpberry maſh; put them both in an earthen pan, and beat it well with a ſpoon till it comes to a cream, or you think it looks white enough, then fill your glaſſes; this quantity will make about a dozen.

O LEMON

LEMON CREAM.

TO a pint of water, add a pound of double refined sugar, and a piece of lemon-peel; set it on the fire to boil, and then let it stand till cold; beat up the whites of six eggs, and one yolk, with a tea-spoonful of orange-flower water, squeeze the juice of four lemons, stir all together, and strain it through a fine sieve into the syrup, take out the lemon peel, and set it over a gentle fire, stirring it one way till it is ready to boil, and taking off the scum as it rises, till it is as thick as cream; rest in a good deal of the peel, and put it into glasses.

You may put in the glasses lemon-peel cut long and very thin.

CLEAR LEMON CREAM.

TAKE a little hartshorn jelly, and put into it the peel of two lemons, taking care there is none of the white; set it over the fire, let it boil, then take the whites of six eggs, and beat them well; take the juice of four lemons, grate in the peel to the juice, let it soak a little while, and afterwards put it together; put in such a quantity of double refined sugar as will sweeten it to your taste; let it boil very fast almost a quarter of an hour, then strain it through a jelly-bag, and as it runs through put it in again, till it is quite clear; after which take the peels of the lemons boiled in it, and put them into a glass; stir it till it is half cold and put it into the glasses.

ORANGE CREAM.

A pint of Seville orange juice, the yolks of six eggs, use but four of the whites, beat very well, strain them and the juice together, a pound of double refined sugar beaten, and set all together on the fire, put the peel of half an orange to it; keep it stiring, all one way; when almost ready to boil take out the orange peel and pour out the cream into glasses or china dishes.

RATAFIA CREAM.

BOIL six laurel leaves in a quart of thick cream; take them out, beat the yolks of five eggs with a little cold cream, and sugar to your taste; pour it into the cream, set it over the fire again and keep it stirring, but do not let it boil; pour it into china dishes, and when cold it is fit for use.

WHIPT

WHIPT CREAM.

UPON the proportion of a quart of very good cream, put a few drops of burgamotte-water, or of cedar, a little orange flower water, and about half a pound of sugar; when it is dissolved, whip the cream to a froth, and take it up with a skimmer; drain it upon a sieve a moment; if for icing let it settle a good while, before you put it in the cups or glasses; continue in this manner to the end, and use what drops in the dish under the sieve to make it froth better; put one or two whites of eggs: any kind of prepared waters may be done with this cream, according to taste and fancy.

CODLING CREAM.

TAKE twenty fair codlings, core them, beat them in a mortar with a pint of cream, strain it into a dish, and put into it some brown bread crumbs, with a little sack, and dish it up, so you may order goosberries.

CURRANT CREAM.

BRUISE currants that are thorough ripe in boiled cream, put in beaten cinnamon, and sweeten it to your taste; then strain it through a fine sieve, and serve it up. You may do raspberries or strawberries the same way. It is best to sweeten the fruit before you put it to the cream, which should be almost cold before the fruit is put to it, else it is liable to curdle.

CREAM OF ANY PRESERVED FRUIT.

TAKE half a pound of the pulp of any preserved fruit, put it in a large pan, put to it the whites of two or three eggs beat together exceedingly well for an hour, then with a spoon take it off, and lay it heaped on the dish or glass

glass salver; with other creams, or put it in the middle bason.

Raspberries will not do this way.

SPANISH CREAM.

TAKE an ounce of isinglass cut small, dissolve it in half a pint of rose water, run it through an hair sieve, add to it the yolks of four eggs, beat and mixed with three-quarters of a pint of cream, two sorrel leaves and sugar to your taste, dip the dish in cold water, before you put in the cream, then cut it out into what forms you please and serve it up.

GOOSEBERRY CREAM.

SCALD tender two quarts of gooseberries, pass them through a hair sieve with the back of a spoon, and to a quart of pulp stir in well an ounce of fresh butter, and sweeten it to your taste; beat six eggs very well, and strain them to the pulp, set it over a gentle fire, stirring it till it grows thick; take it off, and let it stand till almost cold; put in two spoonfuls of the juice of spinnage strained through a fine sieve, and one of orange-flower water, stir it well together, put it into what you please, and send it cold to table.

BARLEY CREAM.

TAKE a tea cup of barley, boil it in milk and water till it is tender; then strain the liquor from it, put your barley into a quart of cream and let it boil a little, then take the whites of five eggs and the yolk of one beaten with a spoonful of fine flour, two spoonfuls of rose water, take the cream off the fire, mix the eggs by degrees, set it on the fire again to thicken, sweeten it to your taste and serve as before.

A STEEPLE

A STEEPLE CREAM.

TAKE five ounces of hartshorn, and two ounces of ivory, put them in a stone bottle, fill it up with water, put in a small quantity of gum arabic, and gum dragon, then tie up the bottle close and set it in a pot of water with hay at the bottom, let it stand six hours, take it out, let it stand an hour before you open it, then strain it and it will be a strong jelly, blanch a pound of almonds beat fine, mix it with a pint of thick cream, let it stand a little, then strain it, mix it with a pound of jelly, set it over the fire till it is scalding hot, sweeten it to your taste with double refined sugar, then take it off, put in a little amber, and pour it into small high gallipots like a sugar-loaf at top, when cold turn them and lay cold whipt cream about them in heaps; be sure it does not boil when the cream is in.

TO MAKE A TRIFLE.

COVER the bottom of your dish with Naples biscuits broke in pieces, mackaroons, and ratafia cakes, just wet them all with sack, pour on a good boiled custard when cold, then a whipt syllabub over that.

TO MAKE RIBBON JELLY.

BOIL two calves feet in five quarts of water, one ounce and half of hartshorn, an ounce and half of ising glass, half a nutmeg, and two blades of mace. Let it boil till it comes to a quart, strain it through the bag, let it stand twenty four hours, then scrape off all fat, put to it the whites of three eggs beaten to a froth; boil it a little and strain it through a bag, then run the jelly into little high glasses, run every colour as thick as your finger: one colour must cool before the other is put on, and that you put on must not be be too hot for fear it should mix. Colour red with cochineal, green with spinnage, yellow with saffron, blue with syrrup of violets, white with cream, and sometimes the jelly itself.

HARTSHORN JELLY.

TAKE care your hartshorn is very good, then take a pound to six quarts of water, let it boil gently till it wastes two quarts, make it a little stronger in summer by adding a quarter of a pound more, take a little out to cool, and if it hangs on the spoon it is enough, strain it off when cold and leave the grounds; then put a bottle of rhenish wine, sweetened to your pallate, with ten cloves, a blade or two of mace, and a piece of cinnamon; beat the whites of eight eggs to a froth, set it over a fire and keep stirring it about; when it hath boiled two or three minutes put to it the juice of six or eight lemons, let it boil two minutes and when it is white and finely curled, pour some

some in your swanskin jelly bag, put a dish under, pour it softly back till it is very clear, then set your glasses under. You make it of calves feet or ising glass.

TO MAKE HARTSHORN FLUMMERY.

TAKE half a pound of hartshorn, three pints of water, boil it till it comes to a pint, and let it cool; then set it over the fire just to melt, take half a pint of thick cream scalded, but cold, a quarter of a pint of white wine, two spoonfuls of orange flower water, sweeten it to your taste, beat it for an hour and a half or it will not mix well, dip your cups in water for it will not turn out well, it is best when it stands a day before you turn them out, stick blanched almonds cut in long narrow bits on the top, they may be eat with wine or cream.

TO MAKE FRENCH FLUMMERY.

TAKE a quart of cream, half an ounce of ising glaſs beat fine: ſtir it into the cream, let it boil ſoftly over a ſlow fire a quarter of an hour, keep it ſtirring all the time, then take it off the fire, ſweeten it to your palate, and put to it a ſpoonful of roſe and orange flower water: ſtrain it and pour it into glaſſes or baſons, when cold turn it out and lay round it baked pears.

TO MAKE FINE SYLLABUBS.

TAKE a pint of rheniſh, half a pint of ſack, ſqueeze in the juice of three lemons, take five half pints of cream, ſweeten it with near a pound of double refined ſugar, put all together, and whiſk it half an hour; take it with a ſpoon and fill the glaſſes, it is beſt a day or two old, but in cold weather they will be good a week or ten days.

LIGHT

LIGHT WHIPT SYLLABUBS.

TO a quart of thick cream put the juice of two Seville oranges, grate the peel of two lemons, put half a pound of double refined sugar pounded; half a pint of sack, put a little red wine and sugar into the bottom of the glasses, some a little sack, and some a little syllabub; then whisk your syllabub up, take off the froth and fill the glasses carefully. They must not be made long before they are used.

TO MAKE SYLLABUBS UNDER THE COW.

IN a three quart bowl put one quart of barrel cyder, and half a pint of brandy, sweeten it to your taste, grate in a little lemon peel and half a small nutmeg, let the dairy maid milk the bowl full, if you have red wine instead of cyder and brandy, put in a quart; and so in proportion to the

the quantity you like to make. It is good with a quart of strong beer, and a pint of cyder.

TO MAKE A DISH OF SNOW.

PUT in cold water twelve large apples, set them on a slow fire, when soft put them on a hair sieve, skin them, put the pulp in a bason, beat the whites of twelve eggs into a froth; sift half a pound of double refined sugar, and strew it in the eggs; beat the pulp of your apples to a strong froth, then beat them altogether till they are like a stiff snow; lay it on a china dish heaped as high as you can, and set round green knots of paste in imitation of Chinese rails, stick a sprig of myrtle in the dish and serve it up.

TO MAKE QUADRILLE CARDS.

TAKE six square tins the size of a card, fill them with very stiff flummery, when you turn them out, have ready a little cochineal dissolved in brandy, strain it through a muslin rag, then take a camel's hair pencil, and make hearts and diamonds; for spades and clubs, take a little chocolate with a little sweet oil upon a marble, rub it till it is fine and bright, if you chuse the suit to be in hearts, you must place the ace of spades first, then the seven of hearts, then the ace of clubs, then the ace of hearts, then the two and three of hearts: if in diamonds the same as hearts, but if you chuse the suit in black then place the ace of spades, the two of spades, and the ace of clubs, the three, four and five of spades. Do the same in clubs: observe that the two black aces are always trumps in any suit. Pour a little Lisbon wine into the dish and send it up.

TO MAKE BLACK CAPS.

TAKE six large apples, cut a slice off the top, put them in a tin and set them in a quick oven till they are brown, then with rose water

wet

CONFECTIONARY.

wet them; grate a little sugar over them, set them in the oven again till they look bright and very black; then put them in a china dish and pour round them thick cream custard.

TO MAKE GREEN CAPS.

TAKE codlings just before they are ripe, green them as for preserving, then rub them over with a little oiled butter; grate double refined sugar over them and set them in the oven till they look bright and sparkle like frost; then put them in a dish, and stick single flowers in every apple; pour round a fine custard. it is a corner dish for dinner or supper.

A FLOATING ISLAND.

TAKE a quart of thick cream, a gill of sack, the rind of lemon grated, sweeten it to your taste,

taste, mill it till it is of a thick froth; then carefully pour the thin from the froth into a deep dish, cut then some french roll, lay a slice as light as possible on the cream, then a layer of currant jelly on that, then another thin slice of roll, then hartshorn jelly, then roll; and over that whip the froth which you save off the cream very well, and lay at top as high as you can. Garnish the rim of the dish with sweetmeats and flowers: it looks well for a middle dish by candle light.

RASBERRY FOOL.

BRUISE a pint and a half of rasberries, put them through a sieve, pound half a pound of fine sugar, and sweeten them; a spoonful of orange flower water, boil two or three minutes, take a pint and a half of cream and boil it; stir it till cold, when the pulp is cold stir them both together

CONFECTIONARY.

ther till they are well mixed, put them in cups or glasses. You make gooseberry fool the same, only of milk instead of cream, and put in three yolks of eggs to a quart of milk, keep stirring till it boils, and afterwards till cold; as the cream and mix the fruit the same only a quart of gooseberries.

Bills of fare for small deserts.

	Moist ananas or pine apple.	
Nectarines.		Walnuts.
Comport of green gages.	Floating island.	Comport of cherries.
Filberts.	Sword knots.	Peaches.
		Bloomage.

CONFECTIONARY.

Bloomage.

Sugar pears.   Nuts.

A basket of fruit.

Green caps   Comport of
                                              green apricots.

A dish of snow.

Almond cakes.   Violet cakes

A basket of fruit.

                                                    Dried
Nuts.   cherries.

Orange tarts.

Strawberries.   Dried apricots.

Jellies.

Custards.   Whip syllabubs.   Quadrille

A middle glass sweetmeats.   cards.

Apple marmalade.   Strawberries.

Royal ice cream.

                                                Transparei

CONFECTIONARY.

Transparent marmalade.

Grapes.		Filberts,
Angelica	Lemon cream,	A cream
tarts.	Sweetmeats wet and dry,	tart.

Crisped almonds and knicknacks.

| Walnuts. | Currant ices. | Figs. |

Mince pies.

| Dried loose bunches | | Chocolate |
| of currants. | | conserves. |

Trifle.

| Almond custards. | Orange flower bomboons. |
| White lemon | Dried goosberries. |

Almond pye.

Apple fritters.

| Almonds and raisins. | Barberry pastils. |

A silver basket with
all winter fruits.

| Bitter almond | Roasted |
| bomboon. | chesnuts. |

Plumb tarts.

A METHOD TO MAKE ALL SORTS OF CANDY.

YOU take whatever sort of fruit you want to candy, let it be orange flower, aniseed, almonds, bits of rinds of either lemon or orange, (which we call zestes of lemon and zestes of orange) sallary seed, powder of coffee, &c. &c. and observe that those fruits must, before offered, be worked as follows, all have been pralined or what is called dry preserved or burnt sugared before as directed. When first thus prepared, you have a square tin box pretty deep, in which four wire grates are made to get in and out at pleasure; you begin by placing one at the bottom of your mould, then you set on it what sort of fruit you chuse to candy, till you have covered all that first grate. Then you place another grate upon that fruit, which you cover the same at the first, then another and then another, till you have thus filled your mould. If you have

not

not fruit enough to employ your four grates, you employ but two, but three, but one even if you can no more, it does not signify a pin, and the operation is in all cafes all the fame. When then all is properly ordered in the mould, you boil in a preferving pan fome clarified fugar till it is to the firft degree, then you fill up your mould with it, or if the mould is not full, you then put only what quantity is requifite to cover what fruit is in the mould; after which, you place that mould in the ftove with a fmall fire for fix hours, after that time you look at your candy if it is confolidate you take it off from the mould, if not, you may let it ftand two hours longer, till it is candied as you would have it: obferve your fire muft always be kept equal, and give the fame heat. Generally there is a little hole at the bottom of thofe forts of moulds which you ftop with a cork, before you take off your candy from the mould you fhould open that hole to let drain all the exceeding syrup: when all is well drained, you put your moulds again in the stove, where there is always the same degree of heat, let it remain there till the next day, when you take your candy from the mould.

THE WAY TO MAKE CARAMEL.

TAKE oranges and pare them, taking off the mere superficy of their peel, without any white at all; then peel off the whole white rind from their flesh, and divide them afterwards rib by rib, set them on a sieve in the stove to dry a little; have the while some clarified sugar which you boil to the twelfth degree, then stick your bits of oranges through the middle with a wooden skewer, and dip them one after another in your sugar, and set them upright on a wire grate at a distance from each other, that they may not touch one another, for they would join together. When your sugar is boiled to the proper

per height you must take it off and dip your oranges as fast as you can.—You may do chesnuts the same way; you roast them in an iron pan, peel them, stick them with the end of a skewer, and dip them in the sugar like oranges.

THE WAY TO MAKE SUGAR ALMONDS, OR FRENCH DRAGEES.

TAKE any quantity of almonds, put them a little in the oven to dry, then put them in the tossing pan with a little fire under, stir them from time to time till they are warm, have then a quarter of a pound of gum arabic, which you dissolve on the fire with a little water; when your gum is dissolved you add to it a little clarified sugar, which you will let boil a little together then put some of that mixture in the tossing pan where your almonds are, and keep stirring till your almonds are dry; when dry, you add a little of your gum to them, and do the same till they

they are dry again, repeating so doing till you have employed all your gum; then have clarified sugar, what quantity you chuse to cover your almonds, to the size and bulk you chuse; boil it to the first or second degree: stir your almonds in till you see your almonds are well covered; you must take care to stir them continually and to keep always an equal fire under your tossing pan; when you see your almonds are well covered, you take a little clarified sugar very light, that is to say, where there is more water than sugar, diminish your fire, and give your almonds three or four washes over of that sugar in moving them, still to make them slip to and fro in the pan; you may even sleek them in the pan with your hand till they begin to be dry; then you continue to sleek them with the pan, then you take them off and set them in the stove to dry.

TO MAKE CORIANDER DRAGEES.

TAKE any quantity of coriander feeds, put them in the toffing pan over the fire, and let them warm; when they are warm throw in about half a glafs of vinegar, then ftir them well till they are dry, then have clarified fugar which you boil in another pan to the third degree, and proceed afterwards for the reft as we faid for the almonds, till you fee your corianders are covered to the fize you want to have them: when that is done, you take your corianders out from the pan, which you wafh well, and when they are well wafhed you put your corianders in again and ftir them well till they are all got warm, then have clarified fugar which you boil to the firft degree; when done you put it in an inftrument of copper, which is made on purpofe for that operation, and at the bottom of which there is a little hole, you hang it up to a pack-threads

ftring

string that your sugar may fall from about a yard height into your pan where the corianders are, while your sugar falls into your pan you keep stirring well your corianders, till you see they are well perled over or rough and grainy like, when they are sufficiently so you take them out and place them in the stove to finish drying them.

TO MAKE CINNAMON DRAGEES.

TAKE any quantity of cinnamon, put it to soak in water for one day, then you take it out and cut it length way in small bits and fine; you put it in your pan and let it get warm, then you take clarified sugar which must be warm and put a little of it in your pan; you then stir it about with your hands, that those bits should not stick to each other till it is dry; you give your cinnamon thus two or three bodies in keeping stirring with your hands till it is pretty well covered; afterwards you continue to add sugar to it it by times till you have brought it to the size you would have it; then proceed for the rest as we said for the coriander, till it is done perling, when you are to put it in the stove to finish drying it.

CARDAMUM DRAGEES.

TAKE any quantity of cardamums, put them in the oven to dry; when they are well dried take them off from the fire, and get all the seed out of them; clean it well, and part all the grains, for they hold together. When you have well cleaned that seed, put it in the preserving pan, and, except the gum, which you are not to put of any, proceed as before directed for the almonds.

CARRAWAY SEED DRAGEES.

TAKE any quantity of carraway, put it in the preserving pan, have clarified sugar, and when your carraway is quite warm put your sugar to it by little and little, stirring it from time to time till you have got it of what size or bigness you please; then go on as we have directed you for the almonds, with respect to the managing of them from that time to the moment of putting them in the stove for drying.

VIOLET DRAGEES.

TAKE one ounce of gumdragon, which you set at soaking in half a pint of water, for twenty four hours; then you pass it through a cloth, and put it in the mortar, first pound it alone to make it whiten, then you will add to it some powdered sugar, and continue to pound it

in

in adding sugar from time to time, till your paste rises very high and stick to your pounder. When you have it thus well pounded, and you see it fastens to the pounder, take it off and put it in a bowl, cut a bit of it and fill it with powdered sugar till you can handle it without its sticking to your fingers, then join to it your violet powder, and take a bit with your fingers, which you roll and dress of the bigness of half a corn of rice; when you have employed thus that bit of your paste which you cut off, you may put the other in a pot to keep it moist, and that which you worked, as we said, you place in the stove to dry, keeping it stirring for fear it should stick one to another, but the fire must be very gentle, when they are well dried you put them in the preserving pan over a slow fire; when they are warmed you put with a spoon some clarified sugar in the preserving pan, and stir them continually till they are dry, then add another spoonful

ful of sugar, dry it again, and repeat so doing till your dragees are brought to the size that you would have them; wherefore proceed as we directed you in speaking of the almonds.

COFFEE DRAGEES.

TAKE the same paste which you saved from the above dragees, fill it with powdered sugar, take some ground coffee which you mix with it, then with your fingers roll some bits of it to the size of coffee beans, put them in the stove to dry, and when dry give them the sugar after the method directed above for the violet dragees.

CHOCOLATE DRAGEES.

TAKE again the same paste as before, fill it with sugar, when done, add some chocolate rasped or grated very fine, and proceed for the rest as for the violet and coffee dragees, except the

the form which you must observe to give round and flat of the size of a farthing or thereabout.

APPLE DRAGEES.

TAKE any quantity of apples, pare them, put them in a pan with a little water, and boil them on the fire till they mash into a pulp; then take them off and put them in a sieve to drain over a dish; when they are well drained pass three or four times the jelly which your apples have produced through a sieve, till it is clear; then weigh it, and weigh likewise a pound and a half of clarified sugar to every pound of fruit, boil this alone to caramel height, then take it off and put in your jelly of apples; set the whole again upon a gentle fire that it may not boil, you skim it well till no more scum comes upon it, then you put it in dishes made on purpose, and let it cool; when it is cold you set your dishes in the stove with a mild fire; when you perceive they have got a cruft on the top, you turn them from the difhes, cut them in four quarters, put them on a tin plate, and replace them again in the ftove to make a cruft on the other fide; when they are well crufted on both fides you fet them on a fieve to dry that you may keep them.

A Method for making all Sorts of Bifcuits.

PALAIS ROYAL BISCUITS.

TAKE eight eggs, break them and put the yolks in one pan, and the whites in another; then weigh half a pound of fugar, which you put in the pan where the yolks are, beat well your yolks and the fugar together with a fpoon, till it makes a white pafte; weigh fix ounces of flour which you put on a white fheet of paper; when your yolks of eggs are well beaten with the fugar, and your flour weighed, and put on a fheet of paper,

paper, take a small whisk, beat well your whites of eggs, till they come up like a syllabub, and they are so hard that your whisk can stand upright in them; then take your yolks which are like a paste, and put them with the whites, and mix them in turning them gently with your whisk. When both the yolks and whites are well mixed, take a sieve, put your flour in it, and sift it gently over your mixture, and continue stirring till you see all is well mixed, and there is no lump of flour in your paste; when your composition is finished, have little paper moulds made long and square, fill them with that paste, and sift on the top of each of them a little of fine pounded loaf sugar, which is called the icing of them, then put them in the oven.

SAVOY BISCUITS.

TAKE fifteen eggs, break them and separate the yolks from the whites, which you put in two different pans; weigh one pound and a quarter of fine sifted loaf sugar, which you put among your yolks, and work well till it comes of a fine white. After which, you weigh three quarters of a pound of flour, which you put on a sheet of paper, and then take your whites of eggs and whip them as we said before. When they are whipped very hard, you will prepare your paste just the same as we said in the preceding article for palais-royal biscuits; for all the difference lies only in the weight of the eggs and that of the flower, which you are carefully to observe; otherwise the way of preparing the paste is all the same. When your paste is quite ready, you take half a sheet of paper, which you place near to your pan, then with a spoon or a

tannel,

tannel, which you fill with paste, you dress your biscuits of what length you please on your paper; and proceed for the rest as before.

QUEEN BISCUITS.

TAKE half a pound of butter, half a pound of sugar, half a pound of flour, quarter of a pound of currants, a glass of French brandy, eight eggs, and a little cinnamon in powder. When all that is properly prepared, take your butter, put it in a pan, and work it with a spoon till it is quite white; then add half a pound of sugar to it, and continue working it the same; when you have worked them both well, add your eight yolks of eggs and the cinnamon, continue still the working of the whole as before; then whip your eight whites of eggs as before directed, and put them in your paste, continuing working the whole together but gently; when your paste is thus well deluted with the whites of eggs in froth, you take a fieve with half a pound of flour in, and fift in foftly over your compofition, mixing it well by ftirring it gently with the whifk: when this is done, take your currants, which you fhall have wafhed and dried by the fire, you will put them in your pafte together, with a glafs of brandy, and mix the whole the fame, by ftirring it gently: then take your tin moulds of whatever form you pleafe to have them, rub them well infide with butter, fet them upon a double fheet of paper, which muft be laid upon a fheet of copper or tin, fill your moulds with your pafte, and proceed as ufual.

RATAFIA CAKES.

TAKE a pound of bitter almonds, pour boiling water over them to rub their fkin off, thed fet them to dry in the ftove, when they are dry pound them in a mortar, take ten eggs, the and ten pounds of powdered loaf sugar. When you begin to pound your almonds, you must put two whites of eggs in the mortar along with them, and continue pounding: in proportion as your paste will dry you will add from time to time a white of an egg: for should you not put whites of eggs to your almonds when you pound them they would oil, which would spoil your paste; when you have done employing ten whites of eggs, and your paste will be very fine, you add to it your two pounds of sugar by little; when your sugar and almonds are well mixed together, take them out from the mortar, and set that paste in a plate, and with two knives you will take that paste and dress it in little flat rounds upon a sheet of paper, and put them into the oven.

ROYAL MASSEPINS.

TAKE half a pound of almonds which you prepare as before; when they are dry you put them in the mortar with a white of an egg, and begin to pound them, adding from time to time, another white of an egg, till you have employed four of them, which is the proportion to every half pound of almonds. When they are well pounded take them out from the mortar, and put them on a sheet of tin; you must take powdered sugar which you will mix with your almonds by kneading it with your hands till you can handle it without its sticking to your fingers; when you have brought it to that point cut a piece of it, which you roll in your hands till you bring it to the size of your little finger, then cut it in bits of about three inches long, and bend them to join the two ends together and make as it were rings of them, continue so doing till you have employed all your paste. When that done, put them in the stove to dry them a little, then you take the white of an egg on a plate, which you whip a little with a fork, then add some powdered sugar till

till it makes a paste, neither too thick nor two liquid, this is what we call *royal icing* when this icing is prepared you take your *massepins* dip them in it, and set them on the wire grate to drain a little, after which you put them on a sheet of paper and put them in the oven.

DIET BREAD.

TAKE twelve eggs, weigh them, and in the other scale put the same weight of sugar, and then of flour. Break your eggs putting your yolks and your whites in two different pans, put in the sugar where the yolks are, and mix them well till it makes a paste very white; then whip your whites of eggs in the other pan, and proceed for all the rest of the preparation with your paste as we directed in speaking of the *palais royal biscuits*. When your paste is quite ready put it in your tin moulds which are made on purpose, some of a pound weight, some half a pound,

pound, and some a quarter of a pound: rub them well on the inside with butter, and proceed for the rest as in page 227.

PUNCH BISCUITS.

Take twelve eggs, their weight in sugar, and half their weight in flour: prepare that paste as mentioned at the article of *palais royal biscuits*; you may only add to it the rasping of lemon peel, which if you do you must add when you are working your sugar along with the yolks of eggs. When your paste is ready, you put it in your tin square moulds, and proceed as before directed.

BLOWED BISCUITS.

PUT the white of an egg in a mortar with the rasping of a lemon-peel, and some powdered sugar sifted very fine; you mix your sugar and
white

white of egg well together with the pounder, adding from time to time a little sugar, till your paste is come to a certain thickness, then take it off, set it upon a tin plate and finish by filling it with sugar, till it sticks no longer to your fingers. When it comes to that point, you take a rolling-pin, you spread your paste on the tin plate till you bring it to half a finger thickness. You have tin moulds of all sorts of figures, some in hearts, some in lozenges, and cut your paste and put it upon paper, which lies on a sheet of tin, and place them in an oven which should not be too hot; the smaller your tin moulds the prettier your biskuits will look.

CHOCOLATE BISCUITS.

TAKE half a pound of almonds, prepare them as we said in page 231, when you take them out of the stove, and they are quite dry

pound

pound them in a mortar with half the white of an egg; when they are well pounded put them on a plate and take two ounces of chocolate, which you melt in a small pan over a very gentle fire; when it is melted put it in your paste of almonds, mixing well the whole with a spoon. When all is well mixed, add the white of an egg and sugar, till you see your paste is a little thick, and that it does not stick to the fingers, then proceed as before.

MILLEE FRUITS BISCUITS.

TAKE any quantity of almonds, prepare them and dry them as in page 231. when dried cut them length way in five bits: take a little clarified sugar of the first degree, throw your almonds in and let them boil one minute only, take them off from the fire and stir them well with a spoon till your sugar is dried into a powder. Then take

take half of your almonds, which are white, away: put a little cochineal to those which remain in the pan to redden them, in setting them a little over the fire to dry the colour, and continue stirring them all the while, then mix the red and the white almonds altogether, take lemon, angelica, and orange dry, cut them in small bits, and mix them with almonds. Have the white of an egg, beat it with a fork, adding some powdered loaf sugar to make a royal paste, let it be very clear, put your fruits in it and mix them well altogether then dress them with your fingers upon paper, making little rock works with them, and put them in the oven.

FRENCH MACARONI.

TAKE a pound of almonds which you prepare as in page 231, when dried you put them in a mortar with two whites of eggs, and begin to pound them; you continue to pound them till you have employed ten whites of eggs, you weigh two pounds of powdered loaf sugar which you introduce by little and little with your almonds, mixing the whole perfectly together, then take your paste from the mortar and put your paste on a plate, and proceed as before.

ORANGE FLOWER BISCUITS.

TAKE twelve whites of eggs and six yolks, observing to let them be new laid; to which add a little rasped or grated green lemon, and beat them all well together; a quarter of a pound of fine flour; when all is properly mixed, bake in proper cases, and glass them as directed for the rest.

BISCUITS OF PRESERVED OR DRIED FRUITS.

TAKE dried preserved fruits, such as apricots, plumbs, oranges, a little orange flower marmalade; pound it and sift it in a sieve; then

mix

mix it with yolks of new laid eggs, and fine powder sugar, till it is come to a supple paste, not too liquid: bake them on paper as the last.

OBSERVATION ON THE BAKING OF BISCUITS.

YOU must take care that your oven should not be too hot for all sorts of biscuits, and above all for those where there are any almonds; because in such a case the biscuits would raise quickly and after they have raised they fall and flatten themselves, when on the contrary if your oven is of a moderate and mild heat, the biscuit dries as it rises, therefore keep it in every stage of its rising, and you have time to give to it what degree of colour you please, either light or deep as you fancy. It is not the same for the biscuits where there is any flour: these require an oven a little hotter than the others, though you must be able to keep your hand in the oven for three or four minutes; the reason why this sort requires

quires a little more heat is, that they have a little more body and strength; it is neceſſary the heat ſhould preſs them a little to force them to riſe. So we ſee that all the experienced and profeſſed biſcuit makers always put firſt in the oven thoſe where there is flour, and a little while after thoſe where there is none, and which are compoſed with almonds only.

ALL KINDS OF ACID PICKLES.

TO MAKE VINEGAR FOR PICKLES.

TO every peck of very ripe gooſberries of any ſort, put two gallons of water, cruſh the fruit well with your hands, and mix it well with the water; let it work three weeks, ſtirring it four or five times a day, then ſtrain the liquor; put a pound of brown ſugar, a pound of treacle, and a ſpoonful of freſh barm; let it work three or four days.

CONFECTIONARY.

days, turn it in iron hooped barrels, let it stand a year or more, it is the best vinegar for use.

OBSERVATIONS ON PICKLING.

BE sure not to use verdigrease, or brass pan, for it is poison to a great degree; for they will green as well by heating the liquor, keeping them on the heatrh.

TO PICKLE CUCUMBERS.

TAKE the smallest you can get, free from spots, gathered on a dry day; put them in a narrow topped jar, put a head of garlick, some white mustard seeds, a few blades of mace, half an ounce of black long pepper, half an ounce of common pepper and ginger, and a handful of salt in your vinegar, pour it upon your cucumbers boiling hot, keep them warm three or four days by the fire, boil your vinegar once every day, keep them close covered till they be a good green, tie them over with a wet bladder and leather.

TO PICKLE CUCUMBERS IN SLICES.

THEY must be large, and before the seeds are ripe; slice them a quarter of an inch thick, lay them on a sieve, betwixt every lay put a shalot or two, throw on a little salt, let them stand four or five hours to drain, put them in a stone jar, and proceed with them as with the small cucumbers.

TO PICKLE WALNUTS BLACK.

GATHER them when the sun is hot upon them, but try them with a pin to find if the shell is hard as they must be soft to run the pin through; put them in cold vinegar with a good deal of salt, let them stand three months, then boil up the vinegar with a little more salt, pour it on the pot; when cold boil them again till they are black,

then

then make a pickle for them thus; to two quarts of vinegar, half an ounce of mace, half an ounce of cloves, an ounce of black pepper, the same of Jamaica ginger and long pepper, a table spoonful of flower of mustard put into a rag, two ounces of common salt, boil it ten minutes, and pour it hot upon your walnuts: tie them down with a bladder they will be fit for use in six weeks.

TO PICKLE WALNUTS WHITE.

PARE the largest French walnuts till the white appears, do not cut too deep for fear of making them with holes, throw them in salt and water as you pare them, or they will turn black, when all is pared, have boiling water with a little salt, put in your walnuts, let them boil five minutes very quick, dry them in a cloth; when cold put them in wide mouthed bottles, and fill them up with vinegar, put a blade or two of mace, a large tea spoonful of eating oil in every bottle,

bottle, the next day cork them well and keep them in a dry place.

TO PICKLE WALNUTS GREEN

TAKE large French double nuts before they are shelled hard, wrap them every one in vine leaves, put some leaves in the jar, then put in the walnuts, take care they do not touch each other, put many leaves over them, fill your jar with vinegar, cover them close that the air cannot get in, let them stand three weeks, pour the vinegar from them put them in fresh leaves, as quick as possible, in another jar, and fill them with fresh vinegar; let them stand three weeks, then wrap them again with fresh leaves, take fresh vinegar, just salt till it will bear an egg, add to it mace, cloves, nutmeg and garlick, boil it eight minutes, then pour it on your walnuts; tie them close with bladder and leather; never leave them open a minute when you take out for use,

CONFECTIONARY.

use, what is left never put in again, but put them in a little boiled vinegar and salt in a small jar.

TO PICKLE SAMPHIRE.

WASH it well in sour small beer, dissolve a little bay salt, twice the quantity of common salt in the beer; fill the pan with the beer on the samphire, cover it close and set it on a slow fire till it is a fine green; then drain it through a sieve, and put it in jars, then take a race or two of ginger, a few pepper corns, with as much vinegar as will cover it, pour it hot on the samphire and tie it close.

TO PICKLE MUSHROOMS.

TAKE dunghill mushrooms, these will not turn yellow at a touch, let them be small buttons, rub them in salt and water with a bit of new flannel, throw them in cold spring water as you do them; then boil them four or five minutes in salt and water, dry them in a cloth till they are cold, put them in glaſs bottles, fill them with diſtilled vinegar, put in a blade or two of mace, a tea ſpoonful of eating oil, cork them cloſe, and keep them cool.

TO PICKLE ONIONS.

PEEL the ſmalleſt you can get, peel and put in ſalt and water for five days, change the water every day, then jar them; pour freſh boiling ſalt and water over them, let them ſtand cloſe covered untill they are cold, let them drain in a ſieve, and bottle them the ſame as the muſhrooms.

TO PICKLE GRAPES.

LET them be large but not too ripe, lay a layer of them in the jar, then a layer of wine leaves, ſo on till the jar is full; take half a pound of common ſalt, half a pound of bay ſalt, boil it

half

half an hour, skim it well, take it off to settle, pour this luke warm on the fruit, lay wine leaves on the top, cover it with a cloth close and set it on the hearth for two days; take the grapes out, dry them on a cloth, but keep them covered; lay them in a flat bottom jar in layers, put fresh vine leaves on the top, then boil a quart of hard water, and one pound of loaf sugar a quarter of an a hour, skim it well and put to it three blades of mace, a large nutmeg sliced, two quarts of vinegar, boil altogether a little, when cold pour it on your grapes, cover and tie them close and keep them dry.

TO PICKLE RED CABBAGE.

LET it be very close, cut it very thin, take cold vinegar, put three blades of mace, some white pepper corns, make it strong with salt, put the cabbage in the vinegar as you cut it, tie it close, it will be fit for use in a few days.

TO PICKLE YOUNG ARTICHOKES.

TAKE them as soon as formed, boil them for two or three minutes in a strong salt and water, let them drain on a sieve, when cold put them in a narrow topped jar, take as much vinegar as will cover them, boil with mace ginger and nutmug cut: pour it on hot and tie them down.

TO PICKLE COLLIFLOWER.

TAKE the whitest you can get, pull them inb unches, spread them on a dish, lay salt over them and let them stand two or three days to bring the water out, then jar them; pour boiling salt and water on them to stand all night, drain them and put them in glass jars, filled with distilled vinegar. Tie them down with leather close.

TO PICKLE RADISH PODS.

GATHER them quite young, put them in salt and water all night, then boil the liquor they laid in and pour on them; cover them close to keep the steam in; when cold make it hot and pour it on again, keep doing so till the pods are quite green; drain them and take vinegar, mace, ginger, pepper, and horse-radish, pour it boiling hot on the pods, when cold make your vinegar twice as hot as before, pour it upon them and tie them with a bladder.

TO PICKLE BARBERRIES.

LET them be maiden barberries not too ripe, put them in a jar with strong salt and water, tie them with a bladder close.

TO PICKLE ELDER BUDS.

GET them the size of hop buds, put them in salt and water nine days, stir them two or three times a day, put them in a saucepan with wine leaves pour the water that came out of them, set them on a slow fire till they are quite green; take vinegar, mace, shalots, and ginger, boil them three minutes and pour it on; then tie them down as usual.

IMITATION OF INDIAN BAMBOE.

TAKE the shoots of elder about the middle of May, the middle stalk, the top not being worth doing; peel off the out rind and lay them in a strong brine of salt and beer one night; then dry them in a cloth single, in the mean time make a pickle of vinegar, to a quart put one ounce of long pepper, one ounce of sliced ginger, a few corns of Jamaica pepper, a little mace, boil it and pour it hot upon the shoots, then stop the jar close, and set it to the fire twenty four hours, stirring it often.

TO PICKLE BEET ROOT.

BOIL them till tender, take the skins off cut them in slices and gimp them in the shape of wheels, flowers, or what you please; put them in a jar and take as much vinegar as you think will cover them, boil it with a little mace, ginger, and horse-radish, pour it hot on the root, it makes pretty garnish for fish or other things.

TO MAKE PICALILLO.

TAKE colliflower, radish pods, white cabbage, cucumbers, or any fruit in season, put them on a sieve, throw salt on them and set them in the sun or before the fire two or three days to dry; when the water is out, put them in layers in a pot, and between the layers put a handful of mustard seed, take as much vinegar as you think will cover them, to every four quarts put an ounce of gumarabick, boil them together, and pour it on them quite hot; let it stand ten or twelve days upon the hearth, or till it is all of a bright yellow, and the liquor soaked up; then take two quarts of vinegar, one ounce of mace, one ounce of white pepper, a quarter of an ounce of cloves, a quarter of an ounce of long pepper, and a quarter of ad ounce of nutmeg beat together; boil it ten minutes and pour it hot on your pickle, with four ounces of garlick peeled.

TO PICKLE NASTURTIUMS.

GATHER the berries soon after the blossom is off, put them in salt and water, change the water once a day for three days together, make your pickle of vinegar, mace, nutmeg, pepper

pepper corns, salt, shalots, and horse-radish, it requires to be made pretty strong, as your pickle is not to be boiled; when drained put them in a jar and pour the pickle on them.

Observations on the Method of making Wines.

TO let your vessels be dry and rinse them with brandy, and as soon as the wines have done fomenting, to close them up.

TO MAKE ORANGE WINE.

TAKE six gallons of water, and fifteen pounds of powder sugar, the whites of six eggs well beat, boil them all three quarters of an hour, and scum it well; when it is cold for working, then take six spoonfuls of good yeast and six ounces of the syrup of lemons, mix them well, and add it to the liquor, with the juice and peel of fifteen oranges; let it work two days and

and one night; then tun it, and in three months bottle it. This wine is stomachical; exhilarates the heart and refreshes the brain.

TO MAKE RAISON WINE.

IN a good white wine hogshead put two hundred weight of raisons with stalks on, fill it up with water, let it stand till it has done working, and put to it two quart of French brandy; when it has done working stop it up, and let it stand six months; then peg it, and if it proves fine, bottle it; then take the lees, distil them, and they will produce you a fine brandy. Raisons of the sun makes a dry wine. Belvidera a fine cape wine. Mallaga a sweet wine; each having a different flavour.

TO MAKE ELDER FLOWER WINE, LIKE FRONTIGNAC.

TO six gallons of spring water put six pounds of jar raisons chopped, and twelve pounds of the best Lisbon sugar, boil all together a full hour, put it into a clean tub till it is cold, then take half a peck of elder flowers, that full are blown, and free from stalks, and put into your liquor; the next day put in the juice of three fine lemons, and a gill of good ale yeast; throw over it a clean coarse cloth, and let it work two days; take the yeast clean off, and put the wine in a vessel; to every gallon add a quart of rhenish or young hock; put the bung on lightly for a fortnight or more, till it has done fomenting, then bung it down close; in six months it may be used.

TO MAKE MORELLA CHERRY WINE.

LET the fruit be very ripe, stalk them, bruise the cherries without breaking the stones; put them in an open vessel together, let them stand twenty four hours, and press them, to every gallon put two pounds of fine sugar, put it in your vessel, and when it has done working stop it close; let it stand three or four months, then bottle it, and in two months it will be fit for use.—This wine quenches thirst, is cooling and good for hot or feverish constitutions.

TO MAKE LEMON WINE TO DRINK LIKE CITRON WATER.

PARE sixty lemons very thin, put the peels into five quarts of brandy, and let them stand fourteen days, then make the juice into a syrup, with

with three pounds of single refined sugar: when the peels are ready, boil fifteen gallons of water, with forty pounds of single refined sugar for an hour, then put it in a tub; when cool, add to it one spoonful of bran, let it work two days, then tun it, and put in the brandy, peels, and syrup, stir them all together, and close up your cask; let it stand three months, then bottle it, and it will be pale and fine as any citron water. It is more like a cordial than wine. This wine is good for young bilious constitution.

CURRANT WINE*.

GATHER the currants when full ripe, on a dry day, pick them from the stalks into a pan, bruise them well with a wooden ladle, let them stand twenty four hours, then run them through a hair sieve, but do not touch them with your hands; to every gallon of juice put two pounds and a half of dry Lisbon sugar,

---

*-Another currant wine, see page 270.

stir it well together, and to every six gallons put a quart of the best brandy, then put it into a clean cask, in two months it may be used, when fine bottle it off.

TO MAKE ELDER WINE LIKE HERMITAGE CLARET.

TAKE nine gallons of spring water, and two pecks of elder-berries clean picked from the stalks, boil them till they begin to dimple, strain off the liquor, and to every gallon put two pounds of Lisbon sugar, boil it an hour, then put it into a clean tub, and let it stand till it is milk warm, make a toast of bread, and spread it over with yeast, put it into the liquor, and let it work for three days, stirring it once or twice every day; then take off the yeast; tun it into a clean wine cask, and to every gallon of wine add a pound of raisons of the sun, (whole) let the cask be full, and let the bung be laid on loosely for two days, then bung it down tight; in four months it will be fit for use; when quite bright bottle it.

TO MAKE AN EXCELLENT BRITISH WINE.

TAKE currants both red and white, goosberries red and green, mulberries, raspberries, and strawberries, of different sorts; cherries too, but not little black ones; grapes black and white; all the fruits must be full ripe, and take an equal quantity of each; throw them into a tub, and bruise them lightly; take golden pippins and nonpareils, chop and bruise them well, and mix them with the others; to every two gallons of fruit put one gallon of spring water; boil all twice a day for a fortnight; then press it through an hair bag into a vessel, and have ready a wine hogshead, put into it an hundred raisins of the sun with their stalks, fill it with the strained juice,

juice, lay the bung on lightly, and when it has quite done hissing and working, put in one gallon of the best French brandy, and stop the vessel close; let it stand six months, then peg it and see if it be fine, if it is, bottle it; if it be not, stop it for six months longer, and then bottle it; the longer it is kept the better it will be; and it is necessary you put in bay leaves with your French brandy.

TO MAKE GOOSBERRY WINE.

BRUISE the ripe fruit well, boil water, put two quarts warm to every gallon of pulp, stir them well together, and after a day or two strain it through a hair bag; to every gallon of this liquor put two pounds of Lisbon sugar, put it in a cask, bung it down close, and let stand for two months; if clear, bottle it, put in every bottle a lump of loaf sugar. This wine creates an appetite, and is of a cooling nature.

HOW TO MAKE FONTINIAC MEAD.

FIFTY pounds of honey, and fifty pounds of Belvidera raisins, fifty gallons of water; boil these fifteen minutes, keeping it well skimed; pour it in the working tub, and put to it a pint of ale yeast, letting it work till the yeast begins to fall; when taken clear off tun it with the raisins, and throw into the cask a quart of white elder flowers; take care to attend it in change of weather; let it continue in the cask twelve months, and then fine it down with wine finings. This wine is good for those who have coughs or phthisic.

HOW TO FINE WINES.

FIX the barrel on a quantity of bay salt upon two boards, the length of the barrel, lay a quantity also on the top, let it stand thus one fortnight,

fortnight, and it will be fine; this clears the liquor better than ising glass, and is neater, being only applied on the outside. All liquors ought to be fined before they begin to fret, or they will not be good. A stone of unslacked lime will keep wine from souring. Observe, when you rack your wines do it when the wind is north, the weather clear and temperate, and to be done in the increase of the moon.

TO MAKE COWSLIP OR CLARY WINE.

SIX gallons of water, twelve pounds of sugar, pare six large lemons, squeeze in the juice, beat well the yolks of four eggs, put altogether into a pot, and boil it half an hour, skim it well as the scum rises; take a peck of cowslips, put them in a tub with the lemon peel, pour the liquor boiling hot, stir it till almost cold; toast a piece of bread brown, and spread it with yeast,

put

put it in your wine and work it for three days, strain it off and squeeze the flowers very dry, run it through a bag, tun it in a cask, lay the bung on loosely for four days; if it does not ferment, bung it down tight, and in four months it will be fit to bottle: You may add a quart of rhenish wine and eight ounces of syrup of citron.

TO MAKE SAGE WINE.

BOIL a quarter of an hour twenty six quarts of spring water; when blood warm put twenty five pounds of malaga raisins, picked, rubbed, and shread, add half a bushel of red sage shread, and a poringer of ale yeast, stir all together and let it stand in a tub seven days close covered; stir it once a day, then strain it out, put it in a rundlet, let it work at press four days, stop it up, and after standing seven days put two quarts of fine Malaga sack, when fine bottle it. This wine is very wholesome.

TO MAKE QUINCE WINE.

TAKE twenty large quinces when full ripe, wipe them clean, then grate them till you come to the core, boil a gallon of spring water and put in your quince pulp; boil it gently a quarter of an hour, strain them through a sieve, and leave the pulp dry in a pan on two pounds of double refined sugar, pare two large lemons thin, put in toe peel and squeeze the juice through a sieve stir it till cool, cut a small piece of bread, toast it, rub it with yeast, put in to work it, cover it close and let it stand twenty four hours; take the toast, lemon peel, and yeast clean off, put the liquor in a rundlet, and in three or four months it will be fit to use.

TO MAKE BITTER WINE.

TAKE two quarts of strong white wine, infuse in it, one drachm of rhubarb, one drachm
and

and a half of gentian root, roman wormwood, tops of cardos, centaury, camomile flowers, of each three drachms, half an ounce of orange peel, of mutmegs, mace, and cloves, of each one drachm; infuse all for forty eight hours, strain it, and drink a glass an hour before dinner, this is very fit for people troubled with the gout.

TO MAKE DAMSON WINE.

GATHER your damsons dry, weigh and put them into an earthen stein that hath a faucet, and to every eight pounds of fruit put a gallon of water, skim it and put it to your fruit scalding hot; let it stand two days then draw it off into a vessel fit for it: and to every gallon of liquor put two pounds and a half of fine sugar; let the vessel be full, stop it close, and the longer it stands the better, it will keep a year; the small damsons are the best; put a small lump of sugar in every bottle

tle when you draw it off. This wine is very fit for those who drink much, and of an astringent nature.

TO MAKE GRAPE WINE.

BRUISE your grapes to a mash, a tap must be placed at the bottom of the cask, tie an hair cloth over the faucet, and set it running; take out the pulp and gradually press it in a side press till the liquor is drained. Air your vessel with a lighted rag dipped in brimstone, burn it till it becomes dry, pour the liquor in through a sieve funnel to stop the drugs, and put a pebble at the bung hole that it may ferment. When it has thus stood for twelve days, draw it gently off into another cask well seasoned. Stop this as the first, when it has fermented and quite calm cover it up; in this manner with the common white grape you may make good white wine; of the red a claret, you may heighten the colour with brazil

brazil boiled in: about a grain of it and strained very clear. The white grape if not too ripe gives a good rhenish taste as in cooling; the muskadine grape produces a fine sweet wine.

WINE LITTLE INFERIOR TO CANARY, OR AS GOOD.

TO give raisin wine different flavours and colours put a few walnut leaves into your sweet wines, in another a few bay leaves, in another a few elder flowers, to make it like red port take twelve gallons of black wine, two gallons of French brandy, and the rest raisin wine; this will serve for a hogshead: and to make it like madeira, take a walnut peel off the outside, chop and steep it in half a pint of red wine, pour it to a bottle of the dry wine, and so proportionably to a greater quantity.

TO MAKE WALNUT WINE.

TAKE two pounds of brown sugar, one pound of honey to every gallon of water; boil them half an hour, skim it and put in the tub to every gallon a handful of leaves, pour the liquor on and let it be all night; then take out the leaves, and put in half a pint of yeast, and let it work fourteen days, which will take off the sweetness; stop it up in a cask and let it stand six or eight months. This is good for people in consumptions.

TO MAKE RASBERRY WINE.

YOUR rasberries must be dry, full ripe, and used just after they are gathered, in order to preserve their flavour; in proportion to one quart of fruit, put three pounds of fine powdered sugar,

gar, and little better than a gallon of clear water; stirring it five or six tims a day, to mix the whole well together, and let it foment for three or four days; put it in your cask, and, for every gallon put in two whole eggs, taking care they are not broke in putting them in. It must stand at least three months before you bottle it.

Your water should be of a good flavour, for in the choice of that, principally depends the making of good or bad tasted wines. Our common water here in London should remain for a considerable time in earthen jars or vases.

BIRCH WINE.

THE best season for making this wine is, a little before the leaves shoot out; the sap being then both thin and clear; to procure the juice, bore several holes in the body of the tree and put in faucets made of the branches of elder, the sooner you use it the better; when you have

got

got a sufficient quantity of liquor, put to every gallon, a quart of honey, stirring them well together; a few cloves, and some lemon-rind, and let the whole boil for an hour, skimming it well as it rises, let it cool, put in three spoonfuls of new yeast, when the yeast begins to settle put it into a runlet that will just hold it, and let it stand seven weeks, and then bottle it, it will be fit to drink in little better than a month, but may be kept good for two years. Sugar may be used instead of honey, putting two pounds to every gallon.

This wine is wholsome, pleasant, and a very rich cordial; good in curing consumptions, and is particularly serviceable in scorbutic disorders.

ANOTHER EXCELLENT CURRANT WINE.

TAKE a hamper of currants, which you squeeze well through a very coarse sieve; when

all

all your currants are squeezed, measure the quantity of liquor you have got, and put it in a large tub; add to it the double quantity of water; when you have well mixed your water and currant juice together, add thirty six pounds of sugar in the tub, and let it dissolve, stirring it from time to time. When your sugar is well dissolved, have a cask, and fill it with that wine. The next day it will begin to work, then you must be very careful to fill up the cask twice a day, either with some of the same liquor, if you have any left, or with a mixture of water and sugar, till it has ceased entirely to work. Then you stop well your cask, and let it clarify itself. It must stand at least three months in the cask before you draw it.

ON

DISTILLING

IN

GENERAL.

THE mystery which the generality of distillers have affected to throw over their art in order to keep it from the public, has not a little contributed to induce many *pretenders* to attempt an explanation of its excellent qualities; which like *quackery* in physick, not only defrauds us of our money, but what is more valuable, injures our health likewise. It is to destroy such

T   impostors

DISTILLERY.

impostors, that I undertake this small Treatise: the plainest and the clearest account shall be the the only means I will make use of to obtain that point.

I will begin first by explaining what is meant by distilling: how many sorts of distillings there are: what are the instruments fit for that business: what accidents it is liable to: what must be done to prevent them. Then I will point the remedies which may be applied to those accidents when they do happen; and at last I will enter into the detail of the different sorts of liquors, that of their composition and the various ways of preparing them.

I begin then by a plain and methodical account of the principle of that art. I will endeavour to omit nothing of what may serve to instruct completely either the lovers of distilling, or the artists who profess it, and make it their particular business.

I beg

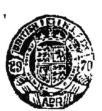

DISTILLERY.

I beg from my readers they will favour me with their reflections and their observations, being always ready to correct myself according to the hints which will be communicated to me for the benefit of the public.

Distilling in general is the art of extracting spirits from bodies.

TO extract spirits, is to produce by means of heat, such an action as will secrete them from the bodies in which they are detained.

If that heat is the proper and natural affection of the bodies, and produces the secretion of spirits without any foreign help, it is called fermentation.

If it is produced exteriorey by means of the fire or other hot matters in which the still is placed, then it is called either digestion or distillation: digestion, when the receipts are

only

only prepared to the secretion of their spirits: distillation when the action of heat has such a power as really to secrete those spirits, and make them to distill.

It is that heat which provoking a commotion and agitation among the insensible parts of any body whatsoever, detaches them, divides them, and procures a passage to the spirits which are concealed in it, by freeing them from the faint or terraqueous qualities with which they were employed.

Considered in that point of view, distilling may become worthy of engaging the attention of the learned, and be the object of their studies.

Infinite are the parts which that art embraces. Every thing which the earth produces, wether flowers, fruits, grains, spices, aromatical or vulnerary plants, and perfumed oils or essences

We shall not undertake to defend its utility nor its charms; it is from the course of this work we hope it may and will be deduced wherewith to make and justify its encomium.

OF DISTILLING IN PARTICULAR.

AFTER having defined distilling in general, we must say something more particular on that article.

They reckon generally three different species of distilling. The first, called distilling *per ascensum*, that is to say by raising, is made by placing the still on the fire or other hot matters, such as gravel, horse dung, boiling water, &c. which promotes a rising of the spirits. This method is the most common and almost the only one distillers put in practice.

6 DISTILLERY.

The second, called *per descensum* that is to say by depressing or defrauding, is procured by placing the fire on the top of the vessel employed in distilling which precipitates the spirits. This method is used by the liquorist distillers but for the oils of cloves, nutmegs, and mace.

Some assert that the oil of juniper berries is very good drawn *per ascensum*.

The third and last called *per latus*, that is to say sidely or by the side is never practised but by chymists therefore we shall pass it over in silence.

DEFINITION OF SPIRITS.

BY spirits is meant the most subtile particles of any bodies whatsover.

All bodies, without any exception are impregnated with spirits in more or less quantities.

All

These particles are an igneous substance, which by its very nature is susceptible of and disposed to a great commotion.

That subtile portion of bodies is more or less disposed to secretion according as the bodies in which it is contained are more or less persons or more or less oily.

DEFINITION OF ESSENCES.

BY essences are meant in distillery as well as chymistry the oily parts of a body: that sort of oil called essence may be extracted from all sorts of bodies and constitutes one of the principles with which they are composed. At least I can faithfully ascertain that in all my operations, it has been my particular observation that I distilled nothing from which I could not extract oil

oil or essence. In every sort of distillation made from fruits, flowers, sweet smelling spices principally and any other sorts of spices put in digestion, I have always seen swiming over the phlegms or faints, a soft and unctuous substance; and that substance is an oil. Now that oil is what is called essence when it is the object of our distilling.

DEFINITION OF SIMPLE WATERS.

BY simple waters is meant what is distilled from flowers and other things without water, brandy or spirit of wine. Such distillations are generally of a phlegmatic quality though fragrant, always charged with the odor of the body from which it is extracted, and even of a more perfect fragrancy than the body itself.

DISTILLERY.

DEFINITION OF PHLEGMS.

PHLEGMS, which some call *faints*, are the terraqueous particles which make part of the composition of bodies; whether this principle be active or passive, I leave to the chymists to discuss I am only a distiller.

However it is, or may be, it is nevertheless very essential for all artists of that profession to be well acquainted with its nature, for many are mistaken in it. Some take as phlegm certain white and cloudy drops which come first when the receipts contained in the still begin to run. Notwithstanding it is certain that these drops are often the most spirituous particles of the matters which distill, which they deprive themselves of very gradually. The whiteness of those cloudy drops is owing only to some moistness which remained

mained in the top of the still; when if they had observed to wipe it off well, they should have seen that the first drop which runs would have been as transparent and brilliant as the last, and it is to their detriment that they throw off those first drops which are the most volatile, and spirituous of their receipts.

Here is an observation which deserves all their attention, and which I recommend very earnestly to any distiller. In all the matters which have first been put in digestion or what is the same meaning, set to infuse the day before, the spirits are the first which fly to the top of the still; when on the contrary in those receipts which have not been set to infuse the phlegm raise first and the spirits afterwards the reason is quite physical and so plain that it requires no farther elucidation to conceive it.

I will

DISTILLERY.

I will add again an observation which I make no doubt will please the curious, and even, I may engage, all those who have some notion of distillery: and though I do not pretend to flatter myself with being the first has made it, I can notwithstanding assure with safety that it has never been mentioned in any book before: this is it. In all the mixt receipts such as would be those in which you would put to distill flowers, fruits and spices together without being previously prepared by means of the digestion; the action of the fire rises first the spirits of the flowers: in such a manner that in spite of the mixture these spirits have contracted nothing from the smell of the fruits nor of the spices. That secretion made, the spirits of the fruits rise next, without any mixture of the spices nor of the flowers. In fine the spirits of the spices came last without the least impregnation of the odour of the flowers nor the taste of the fruits; every article keeps

distinct

distinct by itself in that distillation, and I invite those who might doubt the veracity of this assertion to try the experiment of it.

Another interesting observation I have made on spices, is, that whether they have been put in digestion or not; whether the phlegms or faints have raised before the spirits or the spirits before the phlegms; the spirits you draw from those forts of ingredients are hardly impregnated with the smell and taste of them, and I have always been obliged to mix along with those spirits a certain portion of the phlegms in more or less quantities to give them the taste and perfume of the spices because it is the phlegms not the spirits which contain more of that taste and fragrancy. This observation is absolutely necessary, at least in my humble opinion I judge it such; and may perhaps prove certain satisfactory for a curious reader,

DISTILLERY.

DEFINITION OF DIGESTION.

As the word digestion has often been made use of in this essay, I will not go any farther without explaining what is meant by it and explaining its utility, and even the necessity it is of in many circumstances.

Matters are said to be in digestion when you have them to soak in a proper dissolvent over a very mild heat to soften them. This preparation is requisite and necessary for many sorts of ingredients in distillery. It procures the spirits a more facile issue from the matters where they are contained.

The digestions which are made without any heat at all are those which are more generally used, and the least, because those which are made over the

the fire or by means of hot matters such as dung, &c. in which the vessel is placed, always take away some of the goodness, quality, and merit of the goods, as they cannot but promote some of the spirits, and it is very easy to conceive that this must be so much of the quality.

When you intend to draw essences, the ingredients must unavoidably be prepared by means of the digestion. In order to draw well the spirits and essences from spices, digestion is again there of an absolute necessity. In short digestion enters necessarily in our principles, and is an indispensable one itself.

OF FRUITS AND THEIR DIFFERENT SPECIES.

Various are the fruits made use of in distilling. some are with rinds, some with skins, some kernels,

DISTILLERY.

kernels, some with stones, and others covered over with a shell.

The fruits with rinds such as the *Portugal* orange, as the French call it, or *China* as we call it in England; the cedra, the citron, the *Bigarade* or civil orange, the lemon, and the bergamot are excellent for the liquors of taste, when you make use of the zests of those different fruits to extract the perfume from them together with the oil of essence. The quintessence of those sort of fruits cannot be drawn here as in the countries where they come from; because besides that they lose much of their primitive flavour by importation, the price they fetch in this country renders it an impossible thing for the distiller to think of drawing that quintessence from them with any profit or advantage to himself. We shall speak of the manner of chusing those fruits when we come to speak of them singly. — The bergamot (a kind of of citron) is more commonly made use of for odoriferous waters than for palatable liquors.

Among the fruits with kernels there are few which the distillers make use of except the *reinette apple*, the *rouselet pear*, and the quince. We make what is called *ratafia* or cordial water, with those three sorts of fruits.—But the *rouselet pear* is more ordinarily preserved in brandy. As quince, is fit for a spiritous fermentation, you may distill the spirits on liquor which, by so fermenting comes from it. And the spirit of that water or rather virous liquor is successfully employed in a liquor which in preserving all the delicacy of taste of that fruits acquires its well known beneficient qualities for the stomach.

Cordials are made also with stone fruits, such as cherries, plumbs, apricots, and peaches; these four species of fruits may be preserved in brandy. There are again other sorts of fruits
which

which distillers employ for ratafia and syrups. Such are raspberries and strawberries, which enter in the composition of several sorts of cordials in order to give them a nicer and more exquisite taste. Mulberries, and raspberries, as well as morello cherries are again often made use of to give a colour to certain cordials. There is a syrup made with mulberries and currants which is very agreeable to the taste, and which is very much in use for sick people.

Shell fruits are likewise of great use in distillery. Ratafia may be made with walnuts; and that fruit may also be preserved in brandy when young and tender.

Almonds are made use of for the *Eau de Noyau*. And from that fruit we draw, as well as from nuts, oils for perfumed essences.

We have spoken here but of those fruits which are generally made use of by distillers, there are many others which might be employed with as much success. It is enough to have pointed here the use which is made of them: it behoves the lovers of the art to improve the antient discoveries. The receipts change as the taste changes: but the method and the proceedings we recommend here will always serve and be useful to direct the operations.

OF THE AROMATICAL AND VULNERARY PLANTS.

THOSE plants are called aromatical whose stalk and flower have a strong and penetrating odor though altogether agreeable, such plants preserve that odor a long while after they are gathered even after they are dried up.

DISTILLERY.

Those others are called vulnerary which have an aromatical taste, and which are unctuous and balsamic. We speak here of the vulnerary plants, because we shall give in the course of this work the receipt and method of several vulnerary waters principally that called *arquebusade*. The aromatical and vulnerary plants are in great numbers; but we shall not enter into that detail; we shall content ourselves with only pointing here those which the distillers make a greater consummation of such as melissa, rosemary, lavender, aspic, marjoram, sage, &c. which we shall hereafter give the receipts of. As for the vulnerary they will be found among the receipts which concern them.

From the aromatical plants we draw odoriferous waters, which are exquisite to strengthen the heart and the brain; and which are constantly used in swoons. We may likewise draw quintessences from them which stand in the ſtead of the plants themſelves, in the ſeaſons in which the plants exiſt no more.

Aromatical plants are diſtilled in two different manners; either with water to make ſimple waters; or with ſpirit of wine to make odoriferous waters. Both of them contribute to our health, in contributing to the cleanneſs of the body.

The beſt vulnerary which may be employed are thoſe which come from Switzerland. They generally ſend in thoſe ſorts of plants dry leaves and flowers all together, they preſerve enough of their good quality to be employed here.

The vulnerary plants which enter in the compoſition of the *arquebuſade water*, all grow in France. They are employed in their ſtrength, when they are quite green. It is principally in the time they are in bloſſom, they are to be employed. They may be diſtilled with plain
water;

water; but those distilled with spirit of wine have a great deal more virtue.

Both the leaves and flowers of aromatical plants enter in the composition of the *pot-pourt*. They are likewise employed in the making of sweet smelling satchels, or bags. The general rule is to employ them in their full vigour; and to gather them before the too great heat of the day had deprived them of their flagrancy.

Such is what can be said on aromatical and vulnerary plants. When we come to speak of them in particular we shall enter into a greater detail about them.

Of the various Spices and Seeds used in Distillery.

THE spices mostly made use of in distillery are the clove, the cinnamon, the nutmeg, and the mace.

These four different sorts of spices you may draw by means of distillation, what is called spirits; and by infusion you make tinctures and oils of essence. These spices enter also in the composition of several odoriferous waters, but especially in most of the cordials of which they are material ingredients.

The seeds most known in distillery, are fennel, angelica, aniseed, coriander, juniper, parsely, the carraway, the carrot, and many others. From these various sorts of seeds you draw spirits with brandy for palatable liquors. You may likewise draw oils of essence, or make infusions for ratafias, such as that called ves-pe-tro, or the seven-seeds-cordial.

TO MAKE ORANGE FLOWER WATER.

HAVE orange flower just gathered immediately after the rising of the sun; put both the leaves and the heart of the flower together without picking them in the cucurbite with water; place your still upon the fire in observing well the rules of distillery. Your fire must be here a little quicker than when you distil with brandy, because water being more heavy and less spirituous, it rises with more difficulty, and cannot even rise at all without a quick fire. You must be very attentive upon the quantity of water you want to draw, for should you draw too much, the flower would stick to the bottom of the cucurbite, burn and spoil what is already drawn. Should you draw too little, you would lose what you might get more; forget not to keep your warm tub filled often with cold water; this attention adds greatly to the goodness and quality of the diftillation, and preferves the flavour. The picking of the flowers alone without the leaves, may very well be made ufe of, and the liquor drawn from them will not be in any degree inferior the other.

RECEIPT.

FOR a pound of orange flowers take four quarts of water and draw three.

ANOTHER.

FOR a pound of pickings three quarts of water to draw two, or two and half a pint at moft, in obferving the rules.

TO MAKE THE NEROLY AND ORANGE FLOWER WATER DOUBLE.

THE orange flower water called double, is a water drawn from thofe flowers by means of the ſtill without any water, brandy, or ſpirits whatever, and the method is as follows:

You put in your cucurbite as much flower as it can hold, and place it in a balneo-mariæ, when the heat deadening the flowers by degrees, melts it and ſets it a boiling at laſt; then that is the time that the water called double begins to riſe. In order to make the water as it ſhould be you muſt have flowers freſh gathered immediately after the riſing of the ſun and in fair weather; you muſt make uſe of nothing but the leaves, and pick off all the hearts and hard knobs which form the crown; you muſt likewiſe chuſe the

thickeſt

thickeſt flowers becauſe they produce more in the diſtillation, and have leſs cotton: you muſt keep a pretty quick fire, becauſe this diſtillation is longer than by naked fire, and that your flowers do not run the riſk of burning in the bottom of the cucurbite; but you muſt take care to keep the water of the warm tub very cool, if you will have your liquor of an agreeable ſmell.

Along with that double orange flower water, the neroly or quinteſſence of orange flowers will come alſo; but as this quinteſſence is the oily part it will ſwim at top; that neroly is firſt of a green colour, but after a few days it turns of a reddiſh one. In order to ſeparate it eaſily from the double water, you muſt lay the bottle down, the double water will, when you draw it, come firſt, and the neroly afterwards. Such is the method of making double orange flower water, and to ſeparate the neroly or quinteſſence from it. This water is perfect; very little is required to

give

give a great deal of perfume to the things you mix it with; but the neroly is still infinitely superior to that double water itself, and can admit of no comparison at all; for half a gill of neroly does more than a quart and more of double water; this is a fact which experience will easily convince you of.

RECEIPT.

FILL your cucurbite with flowers to the neck, or less if you want less water; if you will have it good, you must draw but a third part when the flowers are thick, and less if they are not. As for the neroly, its quantity depends entirely upon that of the distilled double water, upon the quickness of the fire, and the goodness of the flowers. The flowers from Provence and Languedoc, give more and better neroly than those of Paris, because the flowers have more strength there.

RECEIPT FOR THE NEROLY.

TO make the neroly or quinteſſence of orange flowers, you muſt, if you want to draw a certain quantity of it, reput your double water in the ſtill, and add to that water ſome more orange flowers; then lute your ſtill well, and put it in a balneum mariæ, under which you keep a very ſmart fire, that the quickneſs of the heat of the common water ſhould provoke more eaſily the riſing of the neroly.

OF THE ORANGE FLOWER WATER LIQUOR.

AFTER having receipts and directions for making ſimple and double waters with thoſe flavours, with neroly or quinteſſence, we muſt ſpeak of another ſort of water made with thoſe ſame flowers, infuſed in ſpirits, and made a palatable liquor; and we recommend our readers

to

to take notice, that this water we are going to give a receipt of, is not to be confounded with the ratafia of orange flowers, from which it differs very much.

To make this liquor water you must first dissolve sugar into fresh water; when your sugar is dissolved, you add to it spirits of wine, and double orange flower water; mix the whole well together, and pass it through the bag; when your liquor is fine it is fit for use.

You may if you will employ neroly instead of double water; but then you must put in the still some brandy, neroly, and water, still it, and throw what you have drawn from that into your syrup, mix it and pass it through the bag.

You must take notice, that in this operation you are not to still orange flowers with brandy to make a liquor of that, because this liquor would

would never fine down; the spirits would be too much loaded with a quintessence which you could command; and that is the reason why we make use of the double water, and the neroly by preference.

RECEIPT.

TO obtain six quarts of liquor, put three quarts and half a pint of brandy in your still; put likewise three quarts of common water, and half a pint of double orange flower water. If your water is not very strong in flowers, you must increase the quantity of this, and dimish in the same proportion that of the common water.

RECEIPT TO MAKE THE SAME WITH NEROLY.

THE quantity of neroly is twenty drops of it to every quart of brandy, which you put in the still; therefore for three quarts and half a

DISTILLERY.

pint of brandy, you put sixty drops of neroly, then three quarts and half a pint of common water, and a pound of sugar.

OF ROSE WATER.

YOU must gather your roses immediately after the rising of the sun, because later the too great heat dissipates their perfume; but immediately after the rising of the sun they preserve still a spirit from the air, which the dew of the night has impregnated them with, and which constitutes their virtue.

You must not gather them in rainy weather, because the rain moistens them, and takes off part of their virtue and perfume.

To make the simple rose water, you only pick all the leaves from the roses, pound them in a mortar, fill up your cucurbite to the neck, and ſtill your water by means of the balneum mariæ, in which you place your cucurbite.

To improve it and give it a ſtronger perfume, you muſt reput your ſtilled water in the cucurbite with the ſame quantity of roſes prepared as above, and ſtill them as the precedent.

TO HAVE QUINTESSENCE OF ROSES.

TAKE the pale double roſe, cultivated in gardens, gathered immediately after the riſing of the ſun; you muſt make uſe of a glaſs ſtill, then you lay a bed of flowers and a bed of ſalt, continuing thus till you have filled the cucurbitic to the neck; when you have preſſed them well, cover them with the top, lute it and ſtop the worm; in that condition you will let the whole reſt two whole days, in order to give the quinteſſence time to come off from the flowers.

It is the salt which makes that quintessence come out of the roses, because they have not strength enough to throw it off them; and without salt, would send up but rose water; but the salt giving them some strength in the space of two days, that they are left in digestion, sends up the oily part of the roses, which is the true quintessence of roses.—After the time prescribed for the fermentation, you set your roses a distilling; what comes first being nothing but phlegm, you throw it off; then luting the recipient to the worm, what comes next is the double water and the quintessence; you separate this quintessence from the water as the neroly of the orange flower water.

The quintessence of rose is not yet known enough to be much in fashion, but if once it takes, its reign will be of long duration. The merit of roses is too well known not to hope a happy succefs from the diftilling of its quinteffence, and the diftiller who will make it well, will draw a great advantage of it befides honour.

OF LILY WATER.

THIS flower is very good to make ufe of, the perfumer employs it with fuccefs for powders, oils, and effences; the diftiller turns it into liquor, fimple and double water, and quinteffence.

TO MAKE LILY WATER LIQUOR.

CHUSE fine lilies, thick and well blown, not at all faded nor begun to decay; you will get thofe flowers as well as all thofe you employ immediately after the rifing of the fun; you will cut nothing but the ftalk of the flower, becaufe it would give to your diftillation a tafte of green; you will leave the flower whole, you will put it in the cucurbite with common water and brandy in the proportion hereafter mentioned in the receipt; you will diftil it upon a naked fire a little quick.

When your fpirits are drawn you melt fugar in water; when melted, you mix your fpirits of lilies with it; pafs the whole through a bag, and when fined down, your liquor will be fit for ufe.

A RECEIPT FOR THE COMMON SORT OF LIQUOR.

THREE quarts of brandy, half a pound of lily flowers, three quarts of water, and a pound of fugar for the fyrup; the whole muft make up five quarts of liquor in all when finifhed.

A RECEIPT FOR THE DOUBLE LIQUOR.

HALF a pound of flowers, three quarts of brandy, for the syrup three pounds of sugar in two quarts of common water; to produce four quarts of liquor in all when done.

TO MAKE SIMPLE AND DOUBLE LILY WATER.

TO make the lily water simple, take good flowers with the above described qualities; fill up your cucurbite and put only common water.

Distil this receipt upon a naked fire, and a little quick, because water rises more difficultly than spirits; observe not to draw too much for fear the flowers burning in the bottom should spoil what has been drawn before; keep your worm tub very cool to preserve the odour.

RECEIPT.

FOR three quarts of common water take a pound of flowers; for more keep the same proportion.

TO MAKE THE DOUBLE WATER AND THE QUINTESSENCE.

FILL the cucurbite of a glass still with flowers to the neck, put less if you want less; place your still in a balneum mariæ, and put no water with the flowers; you will draw by that means a lily water pure very fit for the preservation of the skin. If the season proves very warm you may draw from that distillation a quintessence in the same manner as you draw the neroly from the orange flowers; if you want to draw your water double, draw but the fourth part; and as for the quintessence, as it will swim over, you may draw it as the neroly by inclination, which will let the water run first and the quinteſſence laſt.

OF CARNATION WATER.

THE carnations which the diſtillers employ are thoſe ſmall ones, which, as they ſerve for nothing elſe but the making of liquors, for that reaſon called ratafia carnation. This ſmall carnation has but four leaves; to chuſe it well it muſt be of a dark red, drawing upon black, and of a fine bloomy look; the time of gathering it muſt be in warm weather: this ſort of carnation blows three times a year; it is thoſe of the firſt blowing you muſt chuſe as they have more ſtrength and contain more perfume than thoſe which come after.

Pick well all the leaves from their ſtalk and put them in a pitcher; then pour brandy over them

DISTILLERY.

them, and let them infuse thus the space of six weeks, with a few cloves to help the taste of the flowers.

After the six weeks are elapsed you pass the whole through a sieve and let the flowers drain well, you may even press them if you please; then melt sugar in fresh water and when it is melted mix it with your infusion of carnations. When all is well mixed syrup and infusion together, you pass it through the bag and when fined down your carnation water is fit for use.

RECEIPT.

INFUSION of carnations and syrup half and half. Six ounces of sugar to every quart of water for the syrup, and carnations at discretion for the infusion in brandy.

ANOTHER WAY.

WHEN your carnations are picked as before directed, instead of setting them to infuse in brandy for six weeks; put them to infuse in water upon the fire. In less than three hours your carnations will have stripped themselves of their colour, and be no more but of a pale red as a rag dipped in wine; when that is done pass your flowers in a sieve and press them, then according to the deepness of the tincture you make your syrup. If it is of a weak colour you make your syrup with that very decoction; and if you put as many quarts of brandy as you have of syrup, your liquor will instantly be done, you will not forget to pound a little clove and put it in the infusion.

JESSAMINE

DISTILLERY.

JESSAMINE WATER.

TAKE a quantity of flower of jessamine, which you pick carefully quite clean from all the green stalks and leaves about them, then put them in the still with brandy and common water. That done, place your still upon a pretty sharp fire, and distill your flowers.

Be very careful above all not to draw any phlegms, for you would spoil your liquor which would loose all its perfume; and in the distilling of jessamine it is always the perfume which rises first, when all your spirits are drawn stop quickly your recipient. Then melt sugar in common water; when, done instead of pouring your spirits into the syrup, you will pour your syrup into the recepient over the perfumed spirits. As soon as your syrup is poured in stop it immediately and do not pass this mixture through

through the bag, but the next day to give the diftilled fpirits time to cool perfectly, in order to preferve their fragrance.

RECEIPT FOR SIX QUARTS.

FLOWER of jeffamine fix ounces; three quarts and a gill of brandy and a pint of water one pound of fugar diffolved in three quarts and half a pint of water to make the fyrup.

A BETTER WAY.

TO make your jeffamine-water fine and rich, you will take four quarts of brandy, a pint of water, and four pounds of fugar, two quarts and a pint and half a gill of water for the fyrup, and eight ounces of jeffamine.

ANOTHER WAY.

TO make your liquor fine and dry in the mouth, you will take four quarts of brandy a
pint

DISTILLERY.

pint of water for the syrup, two quarts of water and two pounds of sugar, and ten ounces of jessamine.

ANOTHER WAY.

YOU may set to infuse for a month eight ounces of jessamine in the spirit of three quarts and half a pint of brandy; when that time is elapsed make your syrup, and add half a pint of brandy more on account of the weakening of the spirits, which the infusion of the flowers shall have occasioned, your liquor will be perfect, this method is the best of all.

VIOLET WATER.

THE single violet which comes in the spring is infinitely preferable to the double, and that which comes in autumn. It is then that you must employ what we are going to speak of.

When

When you have picked them clean from the stalks you set them to infuse in brandy or spirit of wine for a month, after that time you will pass your infusion in a sieve, and when passed and you have well drained the flowers; you will melt sugar in common water, then pour your infusion into that syrup and mix the whole well; then pass it through a bag and when fined down your liquor will be perfect and fit for use.

RECEIPT.

THE receipt is exactly the same as that we have prescribed for the carnation-wate. So you must govern it by the same rules and directions except you are not to put any cloves neither whole nor pounded in this, in its stead you will put only half an ounce of new Florence iris. The next of the operation is absolutely governed as in the receipt of carnation water to which I refer.

JONQUILL WATER.

THERE are two sorts of jonquills the single and the double; both blow in March or April, are of a clear yellow between citron and orange, the single are the more odoriferous, the double have their perfume rather more delicate. To make a liquor with it you must proceed as follows.

Chuse jonquills either single or double of the best perfume you can find, pick them and set them to infuse in brandy till they have stripped themselves of their colour. This infusion made, you will melt sugar in proportion of the quantity of the inclosed liquor, and you have passed this through a sieve you mix it with your syrup together and pass it through the bag, then when fined down it is fit for use.

Here

Here is again a better way. Diſtill with brandy upon a pretty quick fire what quantity of flowers you pleaſe, to make ſix quarts of palateable jonquill water, follow in every reſpect the article concerning the jeſſamine-water to make it fine, dry or rich, and as the jonquill will not give its colour to the diſtillation, you will make uſe of the tincture of ſaffron, which you will put in ſufficient quantity to give to your liquor the real colour of the flower, there is no other receipt in this caſe but the good ſenſe of the diſtiller.

You may likewiſe draw quinteſſences from jonquills as you do from roſes, and with the ſame directions, that quinteſſence is good either to perfume other liquors in which you want to give the fragrance and taſte of jonquills, or to make ſmelling waters to perfume eſſences and other things of different ſorts.

F I N I S.

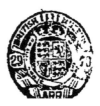

Lightning Source UK Ltd.
Milton Keynes UK
UKHW051910021019
350884UK00009B/163/P